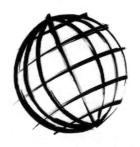

A WORLD WITHOUT CANCER

THE MAKING OF A NEW CURE
AND THE REAL PROMISE
OF PREVENTION

MARGARET I. CUOMO, MD

RODALE.

© 2012 by Margaret I. Cuomo, MD

Rodale books may be purchased for business or promotional use or for special sales. For information, please write to: Special Markets Department, Rodale Inc., 733 Third Avenue, New York, NY 10017.

Printed in the United States of America
Rodale Inc. makes every effort to use acid-free ♾, recycled paper ♻.

Book design by Chris Rhoads

Library of Congress Cataloging-in-Publication Data is on file with the publisher.
ISBN-13: 978–1–60961–885–8 hardcover

Distributed to the trade by Macmillan
2 4 6 8 10 9 7 5 3 1 hardcover

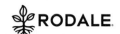

We inspire and enable people to improve their lives and the world around them.
rodalebooks.com

For all those who have lost their lives to cancer—
You are remembered with love.

For all those living with cancer—
Your courage and determination inspire me.

And

For Howard, Christina, and Marianna—
You are my life's greatest blessings.

CONTENTS

INTRODUCTION

Pushed Against the Wall

THE SYSTEM DESIGNED TO STUDY, DIAGNOSE, and treat cancer in the United States is fatally flawed. We would like to think that we have the tools to detect cancer early enough to cure it and that our treatments are safe and effective. We hope people who have dedicated their lives to cancer—scientists in the public and private sectors, oncologists, and advocacy groups—are sharing ideas and data so that, together, they can make progress. We assume that the vast network of government-funded research encourages bold and imaginative new ideas. We trust that compassion, not the quest for professional advancement and profits, is the primary driver of the cancer establishment. Sometimes, all of that is true. Too often, it is not.

For years, I have been observing the "cancer culture" in the United States, and I have become convinced that it is not structured to do what we most need: to determine how to prevent cancer, and then implement our discoveries. Despite decades of promises and a vast amount of funding, the current model of research has failed us. We no longer expect to cure cancer and now talk mostly about living longer with the disease. We are not doing enough to pursue promising new approaches to prevention, and we are not dedicating sufficient energy to applying the strategies that already work.

The good news is that it doesn't have to be this way.

My driving commitment to shift the national approach to cancer from treatment to prevention is at once urgent and personal. *A World Without Cancer* was born through my own life experiences with cancer, as a physician, a wife, a mother, a daughter, a sister, and a friend.

My efforts are inspired by people like Nancy, a smart, savvy businesswoman, a bon vivant, and a generous friend. By the time she was admitted to the hospital where I was working during my medical residency, her breast cancer had metastasized. I still recall the fear in her voice one night as I turned away from her hospital bed. Overwhelmed by the insidious invader that had ravaged her body, Nancy was helpless and hopeless. "I'm afraid. Don't leave me," she pleaded.

It is also to remember Peter. He was a soft-spoken Italian immigrant and a member of my extended family. He put himself through college by working at a shoe factory and went on to build a successful real estate company in New York. For four years, I watched him suffer through treatment after fruitless treatment for colon cancer until he died at the age of 74.

My sister-in-law Penina deserves my efforts as well. Abdominal swelling was her first warning of the peritoneal cancer that would eventually kill her at the age of 47. She combined Chinese herbal medicine with a recommended regimen of surgery, chemotherapy, and radiation, but it proved no match for the disease.

Gregg will always be remembered for his valiant fight to survive lung cancer, accepting all available treatments and their brutal side effects until his death at age 68. His story of courage and hope will live forever on these pages.

My dear friends Alba, Bridget, Carol, Irene, Oksana, and Rosemary and my cousin Nina all succumbed to cancer in their 40s and 50s. Each one of them wanted desperately to survive, and each was a cooperative patient who carefully followed the recommendations of her oncologist. I wish that there had been more to offer them all.

I loved and respected every one of them. I watched their suffering, and I know they all deserved better. They are with me still.

For them, and for Caroline, Joie, Lynne, Richard, Sherry, Susan, Toni S., and many others who shared their perspectives with me as cancer patients, let me be clear: It is time to transform the cancer culture as we know it.

In 1992, I was a young doctor working as a radiologist in the outpatient mammography division of a leading teaching hospital. On any given day, our waiting room was filled with women scheduled for a routine screening mammogram. Among them were patients who needed a follow-up scan because a previous one had shown an abnormality. Others were there because they had felt a breast lump, or their doctors had. Occasionally, a man came in for a mammogram, reminding me that approximately 1 percent of all breast cancers occur in men.

There was always an undercurrent of anxiety in our department, even among the women who were just getting their annual test. Everyone—patients, family members, and doctors—knew that the results of the test could change a person's life in an instant. Understandably, women who had already been treated for breast cancer were the most apprehensive. Nothing was routine about their tests. We were looking for any sign to suggest that the disease had returned, and their fear was almost palpable. That was the situation of a 48-year-old woman I'll call Mrs. Thomson. Two years earlier, she had undergone surgery and chemotherapy for cancer in her left breast. The following year, she received the grim news that the cancer had recurred, and she underwent another operation. Now, six months post-treatment, she had come for a follow-up mammogram at the hospital where I was working. Her husband accompanied her, and from the moment I met them, I could sense their worry. Mr. Thomson, especially, was tense and belligerent. Almost immediately after we introduced ourselves, he told me that his wife had "been through the mill" and that they had "had just about enough" of visits to doctors' offices.

━━━

At that point in my career, I was a seasoned professional, a board-certified radiologist. Not only had I been well trained but I had attended conferences on mammography conducted by world-class, highly respected experts. I understood the science, but I also understood the fear. I tried hard to be patient, sensitive, and empathetic in my interactions with people facing so much uncertainty. It was my goal to treat patients just as I would hope to be treated myself under similar circumstances.

From the beginning of my training, I had been mentored by very attentive and careful radiologists. These doctors always communicated directly and kindly with each patient before they left the mammography room. In most cases, they were able to say that their initial review did not indicate any suspicious findings, while emphasizing that they would review the mammogram more thoroughly and send the final report to the referring physician. Those were the happy times, when the patient would smile gratefully and thank the doctor.

More challenging situations arose when the patient's mammogram did show something abnormal. That's when we needed to draw the utmost from our training and apply our best communication skills and sensitivity. In those moments, I realized that being a really good doctor—a doctor who was effective at communicating with a patient and protecting her interests—had more to do with what I had learned from family, friends, colleagues, and life experiences than with anything I had been taught at medical school.

My mentors were always honest and compassionate in those circumstances. They would look the patient in the eye and tell her that there were a few findings on the mammogram that required further evaluation and follow-up. The term they would use was "suspicious for malignancy." They would never say "cancer," because a mammogram cannot prove that something is cancerous; it can only point to a suspicious finding that requires further evaluation.

Still, when a patient heard the word "malignancy," she would often begin to cry. I became painfully familiar with the look of anguish and the unanswerable question that typically followed: "How could this happen?" Sometimes, a woman would say, "No one in my family has breast cancer" or "I always come for checkups, and I follow my doctor's advice." It was as if we were telling the patient that she was being punished for misbehavior.

Other women had a less overtly emotional response. Instead of tears, some met the news with stoicism and silence. Yet their pained and downcast eyes spoke volumes. I'd watch as a woman left the mammography room wrapped tightly in her own thoughts, and I could almost hear her saying, "Now it is only a matter of time."

As physicians, we are dedicated to easing human pain and suffering, but the realities of cancer sometimes make a mockery of our best intentions. We try to reassure patients, but we are careful not to make empty promises. We'd like to be able to tell them, "Everything will be all right," but tragically, that's not always the case.

An abnormality on a mammogram can turn a woman's life upside down, even if no cancer is ultimately found. At the very least, she will have to undergo more tests, usually with a biopsy as a first step. Depending on the size, type, and location of the suspicious mammogram finding, the biopsy can sometimes be relatively straightforward—a sample of cells can be removed by a radiologist using a hollow-core needle or another technique. If a surgical biopsy is required instead, that will involve a visit to a hospital or an outpatient surgical unit, anesthesia, an incision in the breast, stitches, and a longer recovery.

Regardless of the kind of biopsy, the procedure takes its toll in time and money and even more so in the stress it introduces into a woman's life. If the pathology report says the cell sample is benign, she will likely breathe a sigh of relief, while recognizing the need for more vigilant follow-up. Afterward, her anxiety will linger.

A biopsy result that shows cancer has far greater consequences, of course. At the same moment a woman receives that diagnosis—

perhaps the most terrifying moment of her life—she must also make difficult decisions that involve the treatment triad we currently offer: "cut, poison, and burn."

———

Knowing that Mrs. Thomson had been through all this and more, I was especially patient and attentive as I examined her breasts. As always, I looked for lumps, skin thickening, or nipple changes, any of which would be important clues to her breast health. With the utmost sensitivity, Maureen, the mammography technologist, positioned her in front of the mammography x-ray unit and placed her breast on the cold surface. She lowered the compression device onto her breast, applying pressure to flatten it out in order to capture an optimal view of the tissue. Patients often find this painful or, at the very least, uncomfortable, so Maureen tried to be as supportive as possible as she took the standard x-ray films of the breasts.

Mrs. Thomson and her husband waited as the films were developed and brought to me for review. I stood in a darkroom, secured the films to a light box, and began to examine them methodically and carefully.

Starting at the armpit and slowly moving to the inner portion of each breast, near the sternum or breastbone, I inspected each image for signs of masses, skin thickening, nipple retraction, or other abnormalities. Then I used a magnifying glass to search for "microcalcifications," tiny white specks that signal calcium deposits in the breast. These microcalcifications may be found in areas where cells are dividing rapidly. When they are large, coarse, round, smooth-bordered, and scattered within breast tissue, they are almost always benign. Calcifications that are tiny, tightly clustered, and shaped like commas or flames are more ominous, often representing a malignancy. In postmenopausal women, like Mrs. Thomson, breast tissue tends to contain more fat, or adipose, tissue. Younger women typically have denser breasts. Fat appears dark on x-rays, with white strands of tissue scattered through the breast. This makes abnormal calcifications easier to spot because they stand in stark contrast to the surrounding fatty tissue.

I found nothing abnormal on the film of Mrs. Thomson's right breast. I hoped—and prayed—that the left breast would be equally unremarkable. But as I viewed the outer top part of the left breast, where she had previously had surgery, my heart began to race. I identified a small cluster of irregularly shaped calcifications. Immediately, I compared this area with the mammogram that had been taken before Mrs. Thomson's most recent surgery, and I saw some of the same calcifications. That was a red flag suggesting either that not all of the cancer had been removed or that the cancer had recurred at the same site. I needed a more focused, "coned down" view of the left breast calcifications, with magnification of the area to see them in greater detail.

The technologist courteously and gently asked for Mrs. Thomson's cooperation in obtaining a few more views of the left breast. Mrs. Thomson didn't utter a word, but her husband asked why that was necessary. Maureen replied that additional mammographic views are frequently requested in order to visualize the breast tissue more clearly.

When I received the second set of views, I examined them carefully with the magnifying glass. Again, I compared the new views with those taken previously. My preliminary impression was confirmed: The current mammographic findings would require further attention. Mrs. Thomson would need to visit a surgeon again to determine whether some of the tumor had been left behind in the earlier surgery or whether cancer had recurred in her left breast. It seemed likely that more treatment would be necessary.

I entered the room where the Thomsons were waiting. Mr. Thomson stood with his arms folded across his chest. His wife remained seated. Calmly, I explained what I had found on the mammogram and what it meant—Mrs. Thomson would have to pay another visit to her surgeon.

What happened next is something I will never forget.

Mr. Thomson leaped toward me and pinned me against the wall. His lips, eyes, and jaw held an extraordinary mix of fury, fear, and pain as he shouted directly into my face. "What do you mean? How could this happen? My wife has been through two operations! We were told that it was all out! How could you see more cancer?"

Trying to keep my composure, I said quietly, "I understand that you're very upset and that this is not the news you were expecting."

Mrs. Thomson spoke up, pleading with her husband, "Stop, it's not her fault!"

Mr. Thomson withdrew to his wife's side, but his anguish was undiminished. I sensed, above all, his feeling of hopelessness.

The events of that day were unusual only in the degree of raw emotion that was exposed. Most people do a better job of masking it, but anyone faced with cancer shoulders a huge psychic and physical burden, and every patient and family member will react in a highly personal way.

I never saw Mrs. Thomson again. She may have been treated by her original surgeon, or she may have found a new one. As far as I know, she never returned to our hospital for a follow-up mammogram. However, that searing experience is always with me as I think about the anger, fear, and frustration of cancer patients.

It is an anger caused by having to devote precious time to treatment instead of spending it in the far more fulfilling company of family, friends, and colleagues. It is a fear arising from the assault of an often silent and always insidious disease, one that affects the young and the old, the rich and the poor, the powerful and the powerless. It is a frustration caused by the knowledge that even access to the best treatments, the most accomplished physicians, and the finest medical centers does not guarantee victory against this relentless invader.

Everyone who is diagnosed with and treated for cancer has a unique story. Yet their journeys are also alike in many ways, with a painful and arduous course of treatment almost guaranteed. Together, we can change that, but only if we can first agree not to be shackled by the status quo.

In 1971, when President Richard Nixon signed the National Cancer Act, America declared a war on cancer, and for more than four decades we have continued to wage that war. Think of it: over 41 years battling a disease, with billions of dollars spent to conduct research, build new cancer centers, and develop new drugs and new medical technologies. Still, victory eludes us. In 2012, according to our best estimates, some 1.6 million new cases of cancer will be diagnosed, and about 577,000 people will die of the disease—equivalent to the entire population of a typical American city simply vanishing in a single year. In the United States, cancer is responsible for one out of every four deaths, and the incidence of some cancers is on the rise.

Why have we settled for a medical system that allows cancer to be recast as a chronic and tolerable disease rather than one we should try to prevent? Why do so many scientists at the nation's drug companies and universities turn their backs on the possibility of prevention? How can we transform the agenda?

As I sought answers to these questions from the nation's leading cancer experts, I became increasingly convinced of the need to reset our mission and redirect our efforts. Certainly, we must continue to care compassionately for those who become afflicted with cancer, and we must keep searching for cutting-edge treatments. It is unlikely that we will ever eliminate that need entirely. I am equally certain that we can do more—much, much more—to prevent cancer altogether, or to detect it in the earliest possible stage, when it is most likely to respond to treatment. That's what deserves a far greater share of our funding and scientific talent. That's where we must focus our most vigorous, creative, and bold efforts.

We are all ready for a change in strategy. Many of us have lost loved ones to cancer. Some of us know from personal experience what it means to hear the words "you have cancer." It is time to learn from our success at solving other comprehensive, highly complex problems. After all, we were the first society to reach the moon.

We are also a society that has managed to identify every gene in the human body—some 20,000 of them—in just 13 years, through the Human Genome Project.

We saw what is possible against disease in the late 1960s, when a focused worldwide effort to eradicate smallpox was launched. D. A. Henderson, MD, MPH, was asked by the World Health

Organization to lead this initiative, which included an international assembly of health professionals—Americans, Russians, Czechs, Norwegians, and Brazilians—all working together. The last endemic case of smallpox occurred in Somalia in 1977—10 short years after the project began. In May of 1980, the 33rd World Health Assembly declared the world free of smallpox.

While these scientific goals were different, they shared a mission-oriented, highly focused collaborative approach. The goals were ambitious, the naysayers thought it couldn't be done, and still we succeeded. Why shouldn't we apply this model to cancer prevention?

A World Without Cancer points the way forward. Where I am critical of current strategies, it is because I know we can do better. Where I make suggestions for new approaches that emphasize prevention, it is because I believe they are possible. Where I ask people in every sector of society to act, it is because government, industry, the scientific and medical communities, advocates, patients, and the rest of the American population all have roles to play. I hope this book will inspire a transformation in our approach to cancer.

Dozens of conversations with some of the nation's most accomplished and respected physicians and cancer researchers have confirmed my belief that while we may never be able to cure most cancers once they take hold, we can find ways to prevent cancer altogether, to eradicate it just as we have virtually wiped out devastating diseases like smallpox and polio.

These conversations have given me another reason to hope as well. Researchers who have devoted their entire professional lives to the struggle against cancer, many of then strangers when I called, were incredibly gracious in offering me their time, and they passionately advocated for change. Their dedication and determination are fundamental to the American tradition of accepting a challenge and reaching a goal.

We owe something to millions of cancer patients, each with an ordeal to recount. While we cannot make those precious lives entirely whole again, we can work, for their sake, toward a better future for their children and generations to come.

Reinvigorating our commitment means enlisting the best scientific and medical minds around the world. It means ending the competitive model of cancer research—where investigators hold their findings close to the vest, hoping to publish elegant papers and generate revenue—and replacing it with a commitment to a team science that's dedicated to saving human lives. It means elevating the priority we assign to better nutrition, a healthier environment, pedestrian-friendly communities, and increased physical activity.

With leadership at the federal, state, and local levels of government and a commitment from American people from every walk of life and every part of our nation, we can begin to create a world without cancer.

CHAPTER I

HONORING A
COMMITMENT

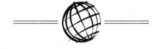

MY FRIEND ROSEMARY WAS 48 WHEN SHE WAS diagnosed with breast cancer. The mother of six children, she was the epicenter of her family, its inspiration and its "glue." She was a partner in every sense to her husband, a well-known author and journalist. Both were passionate New Yorkers, and together they traveled the city's neighborhoods and met some of its greatest characters.

After her diagnosis, Rosemary sought out the most promising treatments from the best minds in medicine. Although the treatments were grueling, she was rarely preoccupied by her own pain and never lost interest in what her friends and family were doing. A woman of remarkable grace and dignity, she maintained a generosity of spirit and usually found something uplifting to say to everyone around her.

I recall vividly my visit to Rosemary's hospital bed on the day I graduated from medical school. She was a patient at Lenox Hill Hospital in New York City, weakened by chemotherapy and swollen from steroid treatments, but when I walked into her room, she immediately focused on me. I had come straight from my graduation ceremony, still wearing my new pink chiffon dress. "It's elegant and simple, just right for this occasion," she told me, as if nothing else could possibly matter more to her right then.

Over the next few weeks, I visited Rosemary several times. The illness had her more and more in its grip, and I was soon doing most of the talking—primarily about growing up with four siblings in the working-class borough of Queens. Rosemary had raised her family there too and was comforted by my stories of familiar people and places.

We could still laugh together, and sometimes we would cry together. She reminded me that little matters as much as the love and support that family and friends can offer.

Still, I was a newly minted doctor, enthusiastic about the great medical advances of Western medicine. I thought surely there should be a therapy or a procedure that could put an end to cancer's ravaging assault. Sadly, I had nothing to suggest.

Rosemary died at the age of 52, with her husband, family, and close friends gathered at her hospital bedside. "She took half my typewriter with her," said her husband at the memorial service. It was an overwhelming, devastating loss, and a sense of hopelessness filled each of us who cared deeply about her.

I was not alone in feeling that I had somehow failed Rosemary. Her husband described the incapacitating experience. "Cancer seeps into your nervous system," he said. "Not the disease itself, but the horror of it."

———

The distress we shared was fueled, at least in part, by disillusionment. What progress have we made since 1971, when our government promised to wage a war that would end in a cure for cancer? Why are we still in a quagmire, without victory in sight? How can it be that in the United States, one out of every two men, and one out of every three women, will develop some form of cancer during their lifetimes? Isn't there something we can do to prevent cancer's relentless march?

In his 1971 State of the Union address, President Richard M. Nixon promised Americans that he would begin "an extensive campaign to find a cure for cancer" and that, in addition to requesting $100 million for that purpose, he would "ask for whatever additional funds can effectively be used." He added: "The time has come in America when the same kind of concentrated effort that split the atom and took man to the moon should be turned toward conquering this dread disease. Let us make a total national commitment to achieve this goal."[1]

The idea made perfect sense. Many experts were confident that if the government marshaled its resources and focused its efforts, we could end the horror of cancer.

After all, the 20th century was the American century, when we could accomplish the unimaginable. Nixon drew resonant parallels. Everyone knew about the extraordinary results of the Manhattan Project, the top-secret research effort that began in 1936 and eventually brought together 130,000 people at 30 sites to develop the most powerful weapon the world had ever seen.

Another outstanding achievement was the first manned flight to the moon. In May 1961, President John F. Kennedy launched the space race in earnest, going before Congress to announce the goal of landing an American on the lunar surface by the end of the decade. We go to the moon, he said in a speech at Rice University the following year, not because it is easy but because it is hard. "That challenge is one that we are willing to accept, one we are unwilling to postpone, and one which we intend to win."[2] In July 1969, American Neil Armstrong took that "one small step for man, one giant leap for mankind."

It showed what teamwork and a sense of urgency could do.

Eradicating cancer was the next logical mission. The disease was taking a terrible toll—although back then we weren't counting cases very rigorously, so no one can be sure just how many people heard those searing words "I'm sorry, you have cancer." By our best estimates, some 650,000 Americans were expected to get that bleak diagnosis in 1972. Two out of every three American families would be affected that year.[3]

We had made so many strides in so many areas of medicine earlier that century, discovering antibiotics to cure infections and vaccines to curb viruses. Surely, ending cancer would be no more difficult.

Our confidence was buoyed by our increased understanding of the links between behavior and disease. Smoking had been established as a cause of lung cancer, raising the possibility that other clear cause-and-effect pathways could be identified.

Treatments were improving at the same time. Nearly two in five people who had received a cancer diagnosis were alive five years later, an impressive improvement over the 1930s, when fewer than one in five lasted that long. Promising new therapies for some cancers were on the market, and others were in the pipeline. Thanks to novel chemotherapy regimens, the three-year survival rate for acute lymphocytic leukemia, a common childhood cancer, had risen from 2 to 15 percent from the early 1960s to the early 1970s. During that same period, the five-year survival rate for Hodgkin's disease had jumped from 44 to 61 percent.[4]

It was time to turn that kind of progress into full-fledged victory. We were moving past some of the research disappointments of the 1950s, when "talk of curing cancer with drugs was not considered compatible with sanity," according to Vincent T. DeVita Jr., MD, a former director of the National Cancer Institute (NCI).[5] Optimism was in the air.

MARY LASKER AND THE BIRTH OF HOPE

Mary Woodard Lasker, a Wisconsin native born in 1900, had a lot to do with kindling a sense of possibility. Jonas Salk, who gave us the world's first polio vaccine, called her "a matchmaker between science and society."[6]

When Lasker first turned her attention to cancer, it was a shameful disease. "Cancer was a word you simply could not say out loud," she recalled. In the 1940s, the family's long-term housekeeper was diagnosed with breast cancer and had both breasts surgically removed. She stoically refused to tell anyone what had happened. That was a watershed moment for Lasker, setting her on a course to change the trajectory of the disease and how we respond to it.

"I am opposed to heart attacks and cancer and strokes the way I am opposed to sin," she declared.

Mary Woodard Lasker was persuasive and passionate in her own right, and her marriage to Albert Lasker forever changed the medical landscape. As president of an advertising firm that marketed iconic American products, including Lucky Strike cigarettes, Pepsodent toothpaste, and Sunkist oranges, he was a man who knew something about the art of selling an idea.

Together, the couple created a powerful lobby that led to huge increases in federal funding for medical research. Mary Lasker's philosophy was pragmatic. "You can solve any problem if you have money, people, and equipment," she declared. Thanks in significant measure to her advocacy, the budget for the National Institutes of Health, the nation's premier research enterprise, increased from just over $3 million to nearly $1 billion in the two decades following World War II.

When the Laskers applied their considerable charm, connections, and business acumen to the American Society for the Control of Cancer, they transformed that institution too. In the early 1940s, it had just 1,000 members, and an annual budget that barely topped $100,000, none of it allocated to research. By 1948, they had taken control of the board, renamed it the American Cancer Society (ACS), and put $14 million into its coffers through aggressive fundraising; 25 percent of those funds were dedicated to research. ACS became an enormously important platform for publicizing cancer and attracting still more funding to combat the disease.

Thanks to the marketing skills of the Laskers, cancer began receiving more coverage in mainstream publications and on the radio, which back then was the news and information mainstay of the American family. It was a time of new openness, a form of "coming out" that changed the national conversation.

With a wave of interest behind them, Mary Lasker and her ACS colleagues lobbied Congress to increase funding for the National Cancer Institute (NCI). Federal appropriations jumped from $1.75 million in 1946 to more than $14 million the following year. The cancer diagnosis of her husband, who died in 1952, added urgency to Lasker's crusade. She found common cause with cancer researcher Sidney Farber, MD, the Boston pathologist who has been called the father of modern chemotherapy. In 1947, Dr. Farber was the first to effectively use aminopterin (which had been discovered by Yellapragada Subbarao, MD) to achieve temporary remissions in children with acute lymphocytic leukemia. The Dana-Farber Cancer Institute, in Boston, one of the nation's leading cancer centers, bears his name.

Convinced that cancer could be cured, Lasker and Farber continued their push for more research dollars, and federal allocations kept growing. By 1961, the NCI had a budget of $110 million.

However, the federal government's commitment was not nearly enough to satisfy Lasker. By the late 1960s, she was calling for a "war on cancer."

She and her allies founded the Citizens Committee for the Conquest of Cancer, which placed a full-page advertisement in the *Washington Post* and the *New York Times* in 1969 that announced, "MR. NIXON: YOU CAN CURE CANCER." The ad also included a quotation from Dr. Sidney Farber: "We are so close to a cure for cancer. We lack only the will and the kind of money and comprehensive planning that went into putting a man on the moon." That remarkable achievement had occurred just five months earlier.

In 1971, Congress held a subcommittee hearing on the National Cancer Act at the Roswell Park Cancer Institute in Buffalo, New York, which had been founded in 1898 as the nation's first cancer center.[7] Representative Jack Kemp of New York put cancer's toll on Americans in stark perspective when he said that the disease had killed eight times as many citizens in a single year (1970) than had died in the previous six years of the Vietnam War. Cancer was the nation's second leading cause of death, after heart disease, and remains so today.

Despite that chilling statistic, witnesses at the hearings were generally determined and optimistic. Scientists spoke enthusiastically about the possibility of conquering cancer. David Pressman, MD, associate director for scientific affairs at Roswell, emphasized that while surgery, radiation, and chemotherapy could be used to manage cancer, the "ultimate goal of all cancer research is the prevention and elimination of disease."[8]

There were vigorous discussions about how much progress was possible until we could answer some very fundamental questions about how cancer spreads. One school of thought was that more knowledge about basic science—for example, about the molecular mechanisms that cause cells to thrive, reproduce, and die—had to come first. Others reasoned that it was not always necessary to fully understand a disease in order to eliminate it. Dr. Pressman fell into the latter camp.

"We have several different causes of cancer. We know carcinogenic substances can produce cancer. We know viruses can produce cancer. We are working on mechanisms for this, but the question of continuing basic research is not a problem," he said.

Dr. Pressman saw basic science and applied know-how advancing together, with each informing the other. "In the space program, the effect of weightlessness on man is still unknown, but that didn't stop us from going ahead and putting a man on the moon."[9]

Thanks in large part to Mary Lasker's advocacy, Congress passed the National Cancer Act of 1971. Two days before Christmas, President Nixon signed it into law, declaring, "I hope in the years ahead we will look back on this action today as the most significant action taken during my administration." Under the legislation, a record-breaking $1.59 billion became available for cancer research over the next three years. A number of other important provisions, which remain in place to this day, stand as testimony to the unique stature of cancer research. The director of the NCI is appointed by the president, rather than by the director of the National Institutes of Health, as is the case at most federal biomedical research institutes. Likewise, the NCI's budget requests are submitted directly to the White House. These factors gave the NCI an unprecedented degree of autonomy and spared it from competing with other scientific agencies to get the largest possible slice of the federal research pie.

At that time, it all seemed very promising. Lasker and her allies hoped that a combination of commitment, resources, scientific talent, and enthusiasm would combine to transform the culture of cancer research. Unfortunately, she did not live to see cancer eradicated. In 1994, her vigorous 94 years of life came to an end due to natural causes. Her hopes for a cure remain unfulfilled.

HAUNTING STATISTICS

More than 40 years after the war on cancer was declared, we know much more about the disease than we once did, but we are not much closer to preventing it. The NCI has spent some $90 billion on research and treatment during that time.[10] Some 260 nonprofit organizations in the United States have dedicated themselves to cancer—more than the number established for heart disease, AIDS, Alzheimer's disease, and stroke combined, according to the *Journal of Clinical Oncology.* Together, these 260 organizations have budgets that top $2.2 billion. [11]

Yet from 1975 to 2007, breast cancer rates increased by one-third and prostate cancer rates soared by 50 percent. Widespread screening with mammography and the prostate-specific antigen (PSA) test played a significant role in detecting these cases, making direct comparisons difficult. Still, we clearly have a problem. Almost 1.6 million people were diagnosed with cancer in 2011. [12] When have Americans ever waged such a long, drawn-out, and costly war, with no end in sight?

One cancer expert has called our approach to cancer "damage control." We deploy the heavy artillery to kill as much of the cancer as we can, hoping that it doesn't escape our weaponry. However, all too often it does. Even if a person is disease free after five years, he or she cannot be considered cured. The enemy may still be lurking. Although some people with a particular kind of cancer will never face it again, others will learn years later that their disease has returned or spread elsewhere.

As of 2009, more than 12 million people living in the United States had a history of cancer—5.8 million men and 6.7 million women. The NCI predicts that by 2020, there will be 18.1 million cancer survivors. [13]

In an ambitious and optimistic moment, the ACS set a goal in 1996 of reducing the incidence of cancer by 25 percent by 2015. The results to date have been discouraging, according to a mid-point progress report published in 2007. [14] The overall incidence of cancer declined by just 0.6 percent a year, well below the pace needed to reach ACS's goal. Just under one in eight American women will develop invasive breast cancer sometime during their lifetimes, according to the ACS. Men have a 1-in-13 lifetime chance of having lung cancer; for women the odds are 1 in 16. (Those numbers apply to both smokers and nonsmokers.) In an aging society like the United States', even this modest improvement may be reversed, because older people are at greater risk of developing cancer.

Meanwhile, the rates of certain cancers are rising, according to the NCI's Surveillance, Epidemiology and End Results (SEER) Program, which gathers statistics on cancer incidence, prevalence, and survival rates in the United States. An upward trend is especially apparent in kidney, liver, and thyroid cancer and in melanoma and lymphoma.[15] The steady increase in the incidence of childhood leukemia and brain cancer since the mid-1970s is a particularly alarming trend.[16]

In more heartening news, there have been small declines in some common cancers since the early 1990s, including male lung cancer and colon and rectal cancer in both men and women. We are also finding some cancers earlier than we once did as a result of more widespread screening.

The fall in the cancer death rate—by approximately 1 percent a year since 1990—has been slightly more impressive. Based on current trends, the ACS has estimated that by 2015, the total number of cancer deaths will be 23 percent lower than it was 25 years earlier.[17]

Still, that's hardly a cause for celebration. Cancer's role in one out of every four deaths in this country remains a haunting statistic.[18]

WHAT'S GONE WRONG?

The failure to realize Mary Lasker's long-ago goal is due in part to the harsh reality that cancer has turned out to be far more clever than we imagined. It is the consummate chameleon, able to develop resistance even to highly toxic drugs. Designed to keep dividing indefinitely, it has an uncanny ability to outwit the therapeutics sent to inhibit its growth. Decades after cancer research began in earnest, Günter Blobel, MD, PhD, who won the 1999 Nobel Prize in Physiology or Medicine for his work in cell biology, told me, "We still don't understand the differences between cancer cells and normal cells."

When the Human Genome Project was completed in 2003, we expected that it would herald a new era in cancer therapy. But Francis Collins, MD, is candid about the practical accomplishments to date. Dr. Collins is director of the National Institutes of Health and previously served as director of the National Human Genome Research Institute. Referencing the hope that knowledge about genetics would transform the practice of medicine, his April 2010 opinion piece in *Nature* was titled "Has the Revolution Arrived?" The answer seems to be "Not yet." Despite the vast scientific information we have collected from genomic research, Dr. Collins called the consequences for clinical medicine only "modest."[19]

We do have a much better understanding of the genetic mutations that raise the risks of certain cancers, which has allowed us to develop some highly targeted treatments that interfere with specific molecules in cancer cells involved in tumor growth and progression. What was supposed to ring in a new era in medicine has instead given us drugs that increase life expectancy for advanced disease ever so slightly, usually by a matter of weeks or months. Achieving even that means using extremely costly drugs that often cause serious side effects.

All that excitement about molecular-level therapies has proven premature, "the goal most challenged by long timelines, high failure rates, and exorbitant costs," writes Dr. Collins. He acknowledges that "the Human Genome Project has not yet directly affected the health of most individuals."[20]

═══

When it comes to treating cancer, we seem to be in a holding pattern. We are still relying on surgery, chemotherapy and other anti-cancer drugs, and radiation, just as we did 40 years ago. "We are stuck in a paradigm of treatment," says Ronald Herberman, MD, the former director of the University of Pittsburgh Cancer Institute.

Today's surgery may be safer than it once was, but in many cases, it still doesn't cure the disease. Cutting out organs and tissues does little to fight cancer's peripatetic capacity to travel through the bloodstream and lymphatic tissue to colonize other parts of the body.

We have more chemotherapeutic regimens to choose from, and we have countless drugs that ease the debilitating side effects of that chemotherapy. Unfortunately, many advanced cancers don't respond to chemotherapy at all. Those that respond do so for only a month or a year or more—and then the cancer often returns.

We have highly targeted radiation treatment that's able to focus beams on the cancerous cells and the tissues that surround them. Ironically, both radiation and chemotherapy can themselves cause other cancers.

Despite their limitations, these treatments do extend the lives of many people, and that has led many physicians on the front lines of patient care to accept cancer as a chronic disease. We think that if we can keep it reasonably well controlled for a long enough period of time, we can proclaim success.

Perhaps the military metaphor, that war against cancer, has contributed to this. Perhaps by lionizing cancer as the ultimate enemy, we have somehow implied that it is a foe too tricky and complex to defeat. We may have created a framework that allows us to declare a stalemate, with no expectation of ultimate victory. We may have put generals in charge who think we should start talking about living with cancer as the "new normal."

At least that is what the director of the NCI seems to be suggesting when he talks about "making cancer a disease you can live with and go to work with." Harold Varmus, MD, who has also served as president of Memorial Sloan-Kettering Cancer Center in New York City, one of the world's great cancer hospitals, goes on to say, "We have many, many patients with lethal cancers who are actually feeling pretty good and are working full time and enjoying their families. As long as their symptoms can be kept under control by radiotherapy and drugs that control symptoms and other modalities, we're doing right by our patients."[21]

But Richard, 58, doesn't feel that way. A husband, father, and businessman, he was diagnosed with a late-stage Hodgkin's lymphoma in 1986 and treated with an intensive seven-month course of combination chemotherapy. "I was considered cured," he recalls.

Twenty years later, he developed abdominal pain, and a positron emission tomography (PET) scan revealed nodes and masses all over his body.

This time, his treatment included rituximab, which belongs to a new class of targeted drugs. Although this therapy was considered a great advance, Richard experienced seizure-like symptoms, accompanied by uncontrollable shaking and chills. Ultimately, he came through the ordeal of treatment to emerge healthy and fit, but no one can assure him that his disease is truly gone.

Ask Richard whether he thinks it is possible to coexist peacefully with cancer. Ask him what he thinks about managing cancer as a chronic disease, as we do hypertension and diabetes.

He won't mince words. "That's nuts!" he exclaims. "What happened to ending cancer?"

An Obvious Omission

What happened, indeed?

Simply put, we have not adequately channeled our scientific know-how, funding, and energy into a full exploration of the one path certain to save lives: prevention. That it should become the ultimate goal of cancer research has been recognized since the war on cancer began. Prevention was certainly important to Mary Lasker when she fiercely advocated for federal funding, and it was an explicit intent of the National Cancer Act of 1971. Yet, we have never fully committed to a concerted national effort to identify and implement prevention strategies.

Not that we haven't talked a lot about it. The ACS has stressed the importance of devoting resources to prevention and to sharing the knowledge we have more effectively. The NCI has its own Division of Cancer Prevention committed to laboratory, clinical, and epidemiological research aimed at reducing risk.

Still, analysts estimate that only about 2 percent of the NCI's total annual budget of approximately $5 billion is dedicated to prevention and early detection.[22] Just 2 percent to the most cost-effective and humane strategy we have?

When I look at the NCI's budget request for fiscal year 2012, I'm deeply disappointed, though past experience tells me I shouldn't be surprised. It is business as usual at the nation's foremost cancer research establishment. The vast majority of the funds will go to understanding the mechanisms and causes of cancer—more than $2 billion is requested for those two areas. It's fascinating basic science, and valuable information may result from this research, but it's not targeted specifically toward the eradication of cancer. Another $1.3 billion is requested for treatment.

And cancer prevention and control? It gets $232 million altogether.[23] Remarkably, in the very same budget report, without any acknowledgment of the contradiction, the NCI states, "Much of the progress against cancer in recent decades has stemmed from successes in the areas of prevention and control."

The failure to give prevention its due has been a long-standing complaint. Political tensions arose in the 1960s and 1970s between those who wanted more attention placed on preventing cancer by addressing occupational and environmental factors and those who wanted to focus on cancer control through treatment.

Scholars at UCLA complained in the *Journal of the American Medical Association* in 1988 that biomedical research, with its clinical and laboratory emphasis, dominated the allocation of federal resources, at the expense of preventive medicine. They called prevention "the most neglected element" of the NCI's efforts to date.[24]

In 2006, participants at a Cancer Prevention Research Summit, organized by the advocacy group C-Change, listed dozens of obstacles to cancer prevention research. Among them are scientific and regulatory barriers to the development of effective prevention therapy; patient and public perception barriers to participation in clinical trials and compliance with drug regimens; insurance policy and practice barriers that affect reimbursement; and intellectual property barriers that interfere with research and development.[25]

Decade after decade, similar complaints have been made, and decade after decade, little changes. It doesn't take great scientific expertise to recognize that prevention is the optimum goal. Dr. Herberman only states the obvious when he says, "Treatments for advanced cancer are more difficult and complex. Prevention has the greatest prospect for progress, rather than waiting until people have advanced cancer that has spread."

Even if cancer weren't so laden with physical and emotional burdens, its costs are rapidly becoming unaffordable. In 2010, total costs for medical expenditures associated with cancer were an estimated $124.6 billion. By 2020, that figure may reach anywhere from $158 billion to $207 billion.[26]

Even with a new commitment in funding and expertise, the prevention of cancer will be a formidable goal.

"Cancer is very hard to tame," acknowledges Eric Ding, PhD, a nutritionist and an epidemiologist on the faculty of Harvard Medical School and founder of the Campaign for Cancer Prevention.

Conducting cancer prevention studies is also expensive and time-consuming. Cancers develop slowly, over many years, so evaluating the impact of preventive strategies can take decades.

"It's simpler to direct research to therapy, rather than prevention," says Larry Norton, MD, medical director of the Evelyn H. Lauder Breast Center at Memorial Sloan-Kettering. "You see activity [against cancer] faster in treatment than in prevention."

Dr. Norton, a proponent of cancer prevention through nutrition, lifestyle, and more research, certainly isn't arguing that a treatment focus is the right way to go, but he does understand why results-oriented scientists are more attracted to it.

Important though research funding for prevention is, resources alone are no guarantee of success. "No matter how much money you have, you don't have a clear path to victory," says Barnett Kramer, MD, MPH, director of the NCI's Division of Cancer Prevention. "It is not just a resource problem. It is not a simple matter—that if we had enough money, we could rid the world of cancer. It is not linear in that we know exactly the path to follow. Progress can't be predicted in terms of where and when the next breakthrough will come."

We can't let the uncertainty discourage us, however. Prevention research will no doubt encounter setbacks and disappointments, and sometimes it will lead us to dead ends. It would be shameful to use them as an excuse not to try harder.

THE WAY FORWARD

Fortunately, there are many promising avenues to pursue. It is time to commit our resources to more aggressively studying the ways in which diet, exercise, supplements, environmental exposure, and other factors can influence the development of cancer. It is time to look more diligently for vaccines and prophylactic therapies, and to do a better job distributing the ones we already have.

We also must get the word out about the prevention strategies we know are effective. As recently as March 2012, public health experts told us that we could prevent more than half the cancers that occur in the United States today if we applied the knowledge we already have.[27] Imagine the transformation that could take place if we showed more respect for the powerful and often-subtle strategies of public health—the ones that help people change their behavior, improve access to health care, and regulate environmental and occupational hazards.

For meaningful progress to occur, scientists, physicians, drug industry representatives, advocates, patients and their family members, and other concerned citizens need to come together in the common interest. We should not "slouch toward a malignant end" and accept cancer as "an inevitability," as one best-selling history of cancer suggests we do,[28] but instead reignite the kind of passion that drove Mary Lasker and her team of indefatigable advocates forward. To galvanize our nation in fulfilling the goal established 41 years ago—the prevention of cancer—we must begin with an understanding of where we are now and an exploration of what is possible.

Chapter 2

UNDERSTANDING CANCER

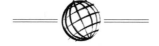

S FAR BACK AS ELEMENTARY SCHOOL, I
thought about becoming a doctor. Fascinated by the
human body and how it works, I read as many books as I
could about medicine and the pioneers who changed the field. I
especially admired Madame Marie Curie, that rare and exceptional
woman of science, for her courage and dedication. When I was
assigned to write a biology term paper during my sophomore year
of high school, I wrote about pathology, the study of the causes and
manifestations of diseases and their effect on people. That interest
led me to volunteer at the pathology laboratory of a busy community hospital in Queens in the summer before my junior year.

Every biopsy performed at the hospital was sent to our pathology lab, which was tucked away in the basement. It was my job to record the name of each patient and doctor, the site of origin of the surgical specimen (such as breast, liver, skin, etc.), and the preliminary diagnosis. A standard black-and-white notebook served as the official log for the hospital's surgical specimens. This was the 1970s, and there were no computers to store data.

During my first week in the lab, I received a plastic bag bearing a tag that read "bronchogenic carcinoma," the medical term for lung cancer—the leading cause of cancer death back then, just as it is today. What I saw didn't look all that ominous. Multiple small masses resembling little gray-white cauliflowers were scattered throughout a healthy, pink lung. Mustering my courage and trying to remain calm, I decided to touch one of the little cauliflowers. Slowly, carefully, I pressed my finger against the plastic bag and felt a hard, unyielding tumor. I still recall my amazement that something so simple and odd-looking could take a person's life.

Years later, as a medical student, I saw cancer cells magnified hundreds of times under a microscope. Irregular in size and shape, they reminded me of puzzle pieces that had been chewed by a puppy and would never again fit together in a smooth, even pattern. When I stained the cells with dye to study them more closely, I could see that the nucleus, which serves as the "central command zone," was often larger and darker than that of a normal cell because it contained more chromatin, a combination of proteins and DNA.

During my surgical rotation in medical school, I often came face-to-face with cancer in the operating room. I saw how a woman's chalky white breast tumor contrasted starkly with the yellowish fatty tissue that characterizes healthy breast tissue. I noticed that the large, bulky tumor of a patient with ovarian cancer contained cystic spaces and projections that looked like polyps. Pancreatic cancer in one man appeared as a gritty, gray-white solid mass within the small, pink, tongue-shaped spongy organ.

Through my training as a radiologist, I became adept at identifying the seemingly mundane spots, lines, and patterns that signaled cancer on mammograms, sonograms, computed tomography (CT) scans, magnetic resonance imaging (MRIs), and nuclear medicine scans.

Breast cancer on a mammogram can appear as a solid white mass, often with jagged, angry-looking edges, or it can look like a star. Thickening of the breast skin, another sign of the disease, shows up as a bright white line outlining the internal breast tissue.

If cancer of the liver is present on a CT scan or sonogram, it may appear as one dark, irregular mass or as multiple dark masses in the normally smooth tissue. Once a contrast agent is administered intravenously to a patient for enhanced CT imaging, the tumors often appear as whitish masses on a CT scan.

Advanced ovarian cancer presents as masses, or "implants," on the liver, stomach, colon, or diaphragm. It may also be visible on nearby organs, including the uterus, bladder, and intestines. Ovarian cancer can cause the abdomen to swell with fluid, sometimes to massive proportions, a phenomenon known as ascites. On a CT scan, this resembles a homogenous gray sea, while on a sonogram it looks more like a black sea.

I soon realized that all cancerous tumors, regardless of their appearance, share the same wild disorganization, distorting the beautiful symmetry and order that typically exist in the human body. I began wondering about the biological process that had transformed once-healthy cells into malignant ones, setting in motion a chain of events that would irrevocably change lives.

Cancer will eventually affect every one of us. Either we will develop it ourselves, or we will travel the rugged journey through treatment with a family member, a friend, or a colleague. Despite the encounter so many of us have had with cancer, there is still remarkable confusion about it. Some patients speak about "the cancer," says David Cooper, MD, an internist who is managing partner of Pro-Health Associates, the largest private medical practice in New York State. "Some people think you can 'catch it.' Or that it happens if you experience a trauma, such as banging your leg."

If people don't have even a rudimentary understanding of what cancer is, we can't expect them to make informed decisions about prevention, screening, or appropriate treatment. If we are to pledge ourselves to eliminating cancer and to building momentum to make that happen, health professionals and educators have a shared responsibility to provide a basic foundation of knowledge to a much broader population.

How Cancer Takes Hold

In Latin, the word *cancer* means "crab." Malignant tumors often look crablike, their irregular extensions resembling crustacean claws. There are anywhere from 100 to 200 types of cancer, and we are still discovering new ones, so that's a very rough estimate. Each is different, depending on where in the body it originates, and each has a unique genetic blueprint. There are five or six subtypes of breast cancer alone.

All cancers have one essential characteristic in common: uncontrolled cell division. "The nature of cancer is that it is programmed for immortality," says Nicholas Vogelzang, MD, chair of the Cancer Communications Committee for the American Society of Clinical Oncology. Normally, our cells grow, divide, and die in a regulated fashion. New cells replace old ones as they age or become damaged. In people with cancer, this balance is disrupted. Though different cancers grow at different rates and respond to different treatments, they share the frightening and uncanny ability to invade and advance through the body.

Cancer does not simply occur spontaneously. For it to take root, a perfectly choreographed process has to unfold. A healthy cell's genetic material must first be altered or damaged, causing mutations that interfere with normal cell growth and division. One theory holds that a single "carcinogenic bullet" may be enough to cause a mutation that starts cancer in motion. Another possibility is that at least two mutations are needed for cancer to occur.

No matter what initiates the process, tumor suppressor genes, which are designed to control cell growth, may stop doing their job. Simultaneously, oncogenes, which are mutated genes that can cause cancer cells to grow, may be turned on. If cells don't die when they should and new cells start reproducing uncontrollably, the extra cells may form a mass of tissue called a tumor.

To understand all this in a slightly more sophisticated way, let's review the basic principles of DNA, which most of us first learned in high school biology. DNA, short for "deoxyribonucleic acid," is made up of four nitrogenous bases that are officially called adenine, cytosine, guanine, and thymine, or A, C, G, and T. These bases are held together by the hydrogen bonds that create DNA's famous double helix structure. Locked in an intricate embrace, these two curving lines contain all the body's genetic material.

The nucleus in every human cell has 23 pairs of chromosomes—very long, thin strands of DNA. Genes are located on our chromosomes, and also come in pairs. We have some 20,000 genes, each coded with a piece of genetic information. Different genes are active in different types of cells, tissues, and organs, producing proteins that affect growth, development, and health.

Cancer can occur when a change, or genetic mutation, occurs in one of the bases in the double helix. The most common mutation is an incorrect base in the DNA sequence—for example, an A base may be substituted for a C, G, or T base. The proper functioning of proteins produced by our genes depends on the accuracy of the base pairs, so even a minor alteration can disable a gene or cause it to malfunction.

Some cancer-causing mutations may be inherited, but about 90 percent are caused by the DNA damage that occurs over a lifetime. All sorts of environmental and occupational exposures can contribute—tobacco smoke, ultraviolet radiation, asbestos, and various air and water pollutants are among the best known. Oxidation, a byproduct of normal metabolic processes, produces free radicals capable of snatching an electron from a DNA molecule. Errors can also be introduced during the routine copying of DNA that takes place during normal cell division.

Fortunately, the body has built-in repair systems designed to interrupt cancer-promoting processes at several points along the way. One backup system mends errors in DNA. Another causes damaged cells to die, an event called apoptosis, or cell suicide. Yet another system puts the brakes on the number of times a cell can divide.

Even if these systems fail, the process by which a normal cell becomes malignant takes a long time, sometimes decades. While family history may increase your risk of that happening, it doesn't necessarily mean cancer is your destiny. Even if you have inherited a genetic mutation, other "good" genes still have to be damaged for cancer to occur.

That means we have many opportunities, at many different times, to intervene and lower our risk for cancer.

———

Cancer often makes itself known in subtle ways. For some people, the first sign is an unusual degree of fatigue. In others, it can be coughing or bloating or shortness of breath, even at rest. Sometimes the signs are more obvious and alarming, such as a lump in the breast that is discovered in the shower, a trickle of blood in the urine, a spot on the skin that gets darker and larger, or a headache that won't ease. Of course, any of these can also be signs of something very different, and perhaps more trivial.

The human body is unfortunately a hospitable place for cancer, which thrives on oxygen and nutrients in the blood. Researchers think it may be so resilient because cancer cells develop a symbiotic relationship with other cells and blood vessels that surround them. A tumor can somehow alter the microenvironment to suit its needs, and in turn, the microenvironment affects how a tumor grows.

Ultimately, the uncontrollable growth of malignant cells overwhelms normal, healthy tissues. Just as a weed steals precious nutrients and water from plants in the garden, cancerous cells can almost literally smother healthy cells.

The greatest danger of cancer is that it will metastasize to nearby or distant sites. One way that cancer spreads is by invading nearby tissues. For example, cancer in one lobe of the lungs can enter another lobe or invade the heart or esophagus. Prostate cancer can infiltrate the urethra and bladder.

Cancer cells can also enter the blood vessels and lymphatic system, circulate through the body, and colonize healthy tissues far from the original cancer site. Various cancers tend to favor specific organs in their metastatic journey. Breast cancer is most likely to metastasize to the lungs, liver, or bones, while colon cancer favors the liver, peritoneum, and lungs.

We use a staging system to determine how advanced a cancer is when it is first diagnosed and as we monitor patients undergoing their treatment. Typically, this coding is a composite measure indicating the size of a tumor or the depth of its penetration through the wall of an organ (T), whether it has spread to the lymph nodes (N), and whether there are any indicators of metastases (M). Each letter is followed by a number—for example, a T2, N1, M0 breast cancer is a tumor between 2 and 5 centimeters that has spread to one lymph node and shows no sign of metastases. Although the TNM system is not used for lymphomas, it is used for many other kinds of cancer.

There are differences in the way that cancers are categorized, even when their TNM designation is the same, but generally, we describe five stages of disease. The earliest stage, stage 0, indicates the presence of abnormal cells that have not spread to nearby tissue and can sometimes be considered a "pre-cancerous" stage. Stage I, II, and III cancers are defined by their particular mix of tumor size and lymph node involvement, and include subcategories (T2, N1, M0 breast cancer is considered an invasive stage IIB cancer). Metastasis indicates a truly advanced cancer and is designated stage IV, regardless of the tumor size. Critical decisions regarding treatment are made according to the staging of the tumor.

THE PATHWAYS TO CANCER

Genetics and environmental and lifestyle choices increase the likelihood of the cell mutations that make us more susceptible to cancer. Those we can't influence—like age and family history—are reminders of how important it is to improve the tools of early detection. Those we do have control over—like smoking, exercise, and diet—are warnings that we need to make a commitment to smart choices, both as individuals and as a society.

Having one or more risk factors doesn't mean you'll get cancer, of course. It just means your odds are somewhat greater than those of someone without them. That can be a powerful incentive for acting on the knowledge we currently have about prevention—and for joining the chorus of advocates who say we desperately need to know more. Risk factors are also a road map of sorts, suggesting the way forward. By indicating where the greatest dangers lie, they tell us where we should focus our scientific resources and what kinds of interventions we need.

People age 65 and older are the most vulnerable to cancer. An inevitable feature of aging is that our backup systems for preventing genetic mutations become less efficient. Since damage to the genes accumulates over a lifetime, being older also makes us more likely to have been repeatedly exposed to DNA-damaging behaviors, agents, or chemicals. While we can't do anything about the passage of time, a better focus on prevention over a lifetime could reduce some of that storehouse of damage.

All sorts of behaviors can heighten risk, or play a protective role. Smoking cigarettes and being exposed to secondhand smoke are certainly prime culprits. Smoking increases the risk not only of lung cancer but also of cancers of the esophagus, larynx, mouth, throat, kidney, bladder, pancreas, stomach, and cervix, as well as acute myeloid leukemia. Almost 175,000 premature deaths every year are attributable to tobacco smoke, according to the National Cancer Institute.[1]

What we eat, how much we drink, and whether we exercise and maintain a proper body weight are other risk factors substantially within our control. Another big category of risk is environmental and occupational exposure, including ultraviolet radiation from the sun, chemical exposures, and ionizing radiation from radon and certain medical tests. Women who take hormone replacement therapy to ease menopausal symptoms also raise their risk for breast and possibly ovarian cancer.

We know something about the biology that explains all this and tells us why it pays to develop the right habits, but we need to apply that knowledge to prevent many cancers. We also need to act more aggressively to spread public health messages designed to educate broad populations and to help change behavior—messages that reach the target audience, respect cultural differences, and motivate people to action.

FAMILY HISTORY

Some cancers occur more frequently in certain families than in the general population. Specific cancers of the breast, colon, prostate, and ovaries, for example, are associated with a "founder mutation," a genetic alteration that originated in a long-ago ancestral chain and has been passed down the line of countless generations.

Some hereditary risks can be transmitted only when faulty

genes are inherited from both parents, while others may exist if just one parent has the genetic defect. Hereditary retinoblastoma, for example, is a rare tumor in the retina of the eye that usually affects children younger than two; it accounts for about 3 percent of all childhood cancers.[2] If one parent has this gene, each child has a 50 percent chance of inheriting it.

One of the hereditary breast cancer risks we understand best involves breast cancer susceptibility genes, known as BRCA1 and BRCA2. The genes themselves don't make us more prone to developing cancer—in fact, they are tumor suppressor genes charged with preventing abnormal cell division and repairing DNA. It is when those genes mutate—and hundreds of possible mutations can occur—that the risk of cancer increases.

Not all gene mutations are harmful. In fact, some mutations are beneficial, and others may be neutral, having no overt effect. We are most concerned with harmful mutations that can increase our risk of developing a cancer or another disease.

Many experts think that inheriting one mutated gene doesn't increase the cancer risk, because genes come in pairs and the normal gene can compensate for its mutated twin. However, women who have inherited a harmful mutation in BRCA1 or BRCA2 are at considerable risk—about 60 percent of them will develop breast cancer and 15 to 40 percent will develop ovarian cancer.[3]

Men can also have BRCA mutations, and those who do are at greater risk of breast cancer and prostate cancer. Melanoma and cancers of the pancreas and fallopian tubes have also been linked to these mutated genes. Both sexes can pass the mutation on to their children, and certain populations are at special risk, including Ashkenazi Jewish women of Eastern European descent.

INFLAMMATION

From the Latin word *inflammare*, meaning "set on fire," inflammation is characterized by heat, redness, swelling, and pain. It is the hallmark characteristic of the body's innate immune response. The first line of attack against an infectious agent, innate immunity is perhaps the oldest component of the immune system, and it has been considered somewhat primitive. In contrast to the acquired immune response, which "remembers" microbial invaders and generates antibodies to fight their return, the innate immune system responds without distinction to all comers.

For years, Gary Stix writes in *Scientific American*, "immunology researchers have paid relatively little attention to this thuggish innate immune system, basically thinking of it as a crew of biochemical bouncers that pummel anything able to penetrate the tiniest opening in a living being's skin or shell."[4]

Inflammation is a sign that the innate immune system is working, first to repel the microbes and then to heal the cells damaged in the process. However, inflammation is also associated with the development of common diseases, including heart disease, insulin-dependent diabetes, and cancer.

"In a blood vessel, inflammation may cause plaque," says Andrew Jess Dannenberg, MD, director of the Weill Cornell Cancer Center in New York City, who researches the link between inflammation and cancer. "In the case of the colon, stomach, or liver, inflammation may predispose you to cancer."

While the possible role of inflammation in cancer isn't fully understood, one theory is that chronic inflammation creates an environment conducive to the growth of abnormal cells.[5] Stix explains that cells ordinarily involved in repairing tissue may be "hijacked to become co-conspirators that aid and abet carcinogenesis. As some researchers have described the malignant state: genetic damage is the match that lights the fire, and inflammation is the fuel that feeds it."

People with chronic inflammatory bowel conditions, such as Crohn's disease and ulcerative colitis, for instance, have a higher incidence of colorectal cancer. Stomach cancer has been linked to inflammation triggered by infection with the *Helicobacter pylori* bacterium. Smokers with chronic obstructive pulmonary disease, an inflammatory disease of the airways, have a higher risk of lung cancer. If we can prove that chronic inflammation pushes cells from a precancerous to a cancerous state, we will be highly motivated to find ways to halt inflammation before a malignancy develops.

THE ROLE OF VIRUSES

The role of viruses in infectious diseases, such as colds, influenza, measles, and AIDS, has long been established, but their links to certain cancers are more newly recognized.

Viruses are the simplest and smallest microbes, containing small amounts of DNA or RNA and enclosed in a protective protein coat called a capsid. Unable to reproduce on their own, viruses infect living cells, inserting their genetic information into the chromosomes of their hosts in order to make additional copies of themselves. While sharing many common characteristics, the viruses associated with cancer "have very different genomes, life cycles and represent a number of virus families," explains John B. Liao, MD, PhD, in the *Yale Journal of Biology and Medicine*.[6]

Dr. Liao emphasizes that viral infection alone does not cause most cancers; some combination of other factors, including the health of the immune system, exposure to other carcinogens, genetic tendencies, and acquired DNA mutations, may also be involved. Nonetheless, an estimated 15 percent of cancers around the world are linked to viruses. These include some cancers of the liver, cervix, head, and neck, as well as certain lymphomas, leukemias, and sarcomas.

For example, hepatitis B and C viruses, which can be transmitted through blood transfusions, intravenous drug use, or unprotected sex, are responsible for 70 to 85 percent of cancers that originate in the liver.[7]

The human papillomavirus (HPV), transmitted through skin-to-skin contact, usually during sexual intercourse, is the primary cause of cervical cancer (it also causes genital warts). About half of sexually active men and women are infected with HPV at some point in their lives. Not all strains cause cancer, and in 90 percent of cases, our immune system will destroy the virus. Still, HPV was responsible for more than 11,600 cases of cervical cancer among women in 2007, the most recent date for which comprehensive Centers for Disease Control and Prevention (CDC) data are available. All told, more than 20,000 women had HPV-associated cancers that year, including cancers of the anus, vulva, and head and neck.

HPV is also associated with more than 11,000 cases of cancer in men. More than 8,500 of these are head and neck cancers in the oropharyngeal region, which includes the back of the throat, the base of the tongue, and the tonsils.[8] About 60 percent of the oropharyngeal cancers that occur in both men and women are linked to HPV.[9]

Vaccines are one of the best prevention tools we have ever developed, but we don't have many of them for cancer, and too few people get the ones we do have. The hepatitis B vaccine, introduced in the early 1980s, has helped prevent liver cancer, but large segments of the population have not been immunized. The HPV vaccine, in use only since 2006, protects against about 70 percent of the strains that cause cervical cancer. It won't be effective in women already infected with the virus, but now that children and young adults are being vaccinated regularly, we can expect to see rates of cervical cancer drop over time.

No vaccines exist for the other cancer-causing viruses. In addition to the hepatitis C virus, these include the Epstein-Barr virus, which is associated with a number of cancers, including Hodgkin's disease; human herpes virus 8, associated with Kaposi's sarcoma; and human T-lymphotropic virus type 1, which is associated with leukemia. This is a promising area for more research.

—————

Regardless of why a healthy cell first mutates, and why the body's defense system fails to stop its spread, one thing is certain: Cancer doesn't play favorites. It doesn't care whether you are Steve Jobs or a city bus driver; whether you are a new mom, a middle-age Little League coach, a World War II vet, or a first grader.

Yet considering the horrific toll it takes, cancer is far from impressive under the microscope, as I first saw in medical school. We should be able to outsmart it.

So many opportunities to do just that lie within reach. First, though, we have to *find* the cancer—and it's a lot better to do that before the cells start to divide in their characteristic crazy-quilt fashion. That's why we are so interested in discovering better tools for early detection.

THE LANGUAGE OF CANCER

Scientists name each cancer after the organ or cell in which it originates—breast cancer, lung cancer, prostate cancer, etc.—and within each organ there are many different subtypes. All told, there are an estimated 100 to 200 different types of cancer, which generally fall into these broad categories:

SOLID TUMORS are masses of abnormal tissue without fluid-filled spaces, i.e., cysts. Solid tumors can be benign or malignant and are named for the type of cells that form them, for example, carcinomas, lymphomas, and sarcomas.

ADENOCARCINOMA describes any cancer that affects a gland (*adeno* comes from the Latin word for "gland"). Thus we have breast adenocarcinoma, lung adenocarcinoma, and pancreatic adenocarcinoma.

CARCINOMAS are cancers that occur in the skin or the tissues that line or cover internal organs. The suffix *-oma*, from the Greek for "tumor" or "swelling," appears frequently in cancer names. A carcinoma can also be named after the cell in which it originates—renal cell carcinoma, squamous cell carcinoma, or basal cell carcinoma, for instance.

LYMPHOMA AND MYELOMA affect the immune system. Lymphoma is a carcinoma of lymphocytes, which are white blood cells found in the immune system. Myeloma—from the Greek word *myelos,* for "marrow"—affects bone marrow.

SARCOMA, derived from *sar,* from the Greek word for "flesh," refers to cancers that develop in tissues connecting, supporting, or surrounding other structures and organs of the body, such as muscles, tendons, and nerves. For example, osteosarcoma refers to bone cancer, and chondrosarcoma affects cartilage.

LEUKEMIA, from *leukos,* the Greek word meaning "clear and white," and *haima,* meaning "blood," is characterized by the growth of abnormal white blood cells—leukemic cells—in bone marrow. Leukemias do not generally form solid tumors.

MELANOMA originates in the skin cells known as melanocytes, which produce melanin, or dark brown pigment. *Melas* is the Greek for "black."

CENTRAL NERVOUS SYSTEM CANCER refers to any carcinoma that affects the brain and spinal cord.

CHAPTER 3

THE PROMISE AND LIMITS OF CANCER SCREENING

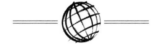

GET YOURSELF SCREENED FOR CANCER! THAT message seems to be everywhere—in pamphlets at the doctor's office, public service announcements on television, and health articles online and in print. Even celebrities are helping to get the word out, sometimes by referencing their own experiences with the disease.

With all that talk, it is easy to make the assumption that every cancer screening is good. The theory certainly seems sound: Screening tests should help to find cancers early, before symptoms occur and before they spread, when they are likely to be easier to treat.

This early diagnosis and treatment is known as secondary prevention—in contrast to primary prevention, aimed at preventing disease from ever occurring, and tertiary prevention, focused on managing disease to prevent further complications or death.

However, the truth about screening turns out to be far more complex than we imagined. Many patients have not been fully informed of the benefits, risks, and uncertainties of these tests, and the value of some tests has been oversold. That doesn't change the fact that effective early detection should be a core component of a bold cancer-eradicating commitment. The problem is that many of our current tools for identifying cancer early aren't ideal.

Even the most widely used tests can miss the presence of cancer. Or, they can find something suspicious, leading to invasive, unnecessary diagnostic testing. Occasionally, cell changes that would never have resulted in cancer are treated aggressively, as if the cancer were already present. That better-safe-than-sorry approach has very real physical, emotional, and financial consequences, which in many cases are not openly discussed.

Such is the degree of uncertainty about screening that one well-respected medical group makes recommendations that are very different from those of another medical group. Patients and their doctors are understandably confused about who should be screened, for what and when.

―――――

As we wade into this murky area, let me underscore the importance of detecting cancer early, before the cells grow or spread. Finding markers that warn us of real danger should be one of our research priorities. With heart disease and diabetes, we know some of the symptoms that precede full-blown disease, and when we detect a risk, we have treatments to offer. We measure blood pressure routinely, for example, and can prescribe a host of effective medications to control it. There is nothing comparable for cancer.

"It's silent, silent, silent and then, boom, you get it. You can have a perfectly healthy 20- or 50-year-old stricken with it out of the blue," says Eric Ding, PhD, founder of the Campaign for Cancer Prevention, which partners with Brigham and Women's Hospital in Boston to promote cutting-edge cancer research and prevention strategies. "I am not sure if we can prevent you from getting cancer at age 80. As we increase longevity, we increase the likelihood of cancer. But we want to prevent you from getting it at age 50 or 60."

That's what our most accurate screening tests help to do. The Pap test, for example, can detect abnormal or cancerous cells at a point when cervical cancer can be completely eliminated or more easily treated.

In 1950, before the test became routine, the Centers for Disease Control and Prevention reported more than 10 deaths per 100,000 white women and 18 deaths per 100,000 nonwhite women due to cervical cancer. By 2007, overall death rates among all women had dropped to 2.4 per 100,000.[1]

Screening for colorectal cancer has also made a big difference. The CDC tells us that from 2003 to 2007, some 66,000 cases of the disease were prevented and 32,000 lives were saved as a result, compared with 2002.[2]

While there is some disagreement about how frequently to administer Pap tests and colonoscopies, there is a general consensus that they work well.

Mammography for breast cancer and the prostate-specific antigen (PSA) test for prostate cancer generate far more controversy and emotion. These tools can't be discarded until we have better alternatives, but they are far from the saviors we once thought they were, and our heavy reliance on them has slowly lost some luster.

My own take is that our most prominent screening tests—for cancers of the colon, cervix, and breast—generally have benefits that outweigh their limitations. Not everyone agrees, and the pros and cons of these tests, and especially the individual risk factors that can influence decision making, need to be explored carefully by patients and their doctors in one-on-one discussions.

Some patients, worried more about missing a cancer than about undergoing unnecessary treatment, will eagerly embrace any screening test available. Others, concerned about the false-positive results that lead to unnecessary and potentially harmful further testing, will avoid them as much as possible. These are reasoned decisions, but if the science were more authoritative, all of us could act on the basis of evidence, rather than on informed opinion and personal preference.

We should expect our scientific leaders to commit themselves to untangling the facts, determining what does and does not work, and finding better ways to screen. The National Cancer Institute (NCI) should pledge to do that, especially when it comes to detecting breast, prostate, and lung cancers, where the death toll is huge and the screening tests far less than optimal.

FEW TESTS, MANY QUESTIONS

There are many reasons why we lack good screening options. Deficits in our knowledge about a cancer's biological pathways, or a difficult-to-reach location, make some tumors hard to find. Sometimes a cancer is so small that it eludes detection, or the interval between tests is too long to catch cancer as it begins to take root.

The criteria for a good screening test are fairly straightforward. To be useful, a test designed to screen a large population of apparently healthy people has to be fairly simple to perform, noninvasive, and affordable, and its benefits should outweigh any potential harms. The test should also be easy to evaluate and accurate at detecting disease, and we need to know how often it should be conducted to give us the best possible information.

The most useful screening tests strike the right balance between being sensitive and being specific. The concept of sensitivity refers to a test's ability to identify people who have a certain cancer; if it isn't sensitive enough, it is likely to miss too many of them. That's called a false-negative result—the test indicates that there is no cancer present when there actually is.

Specificity refers to how well a test avoids tagging someone as having cancer who actually does not. In other words, it doesn't come up with too many false-positive results, which needlessly subject people to more anxiety-producing tests to show they are cancer free.

A screening test with 100 percent sensitivity and specificity is the ultimate goal, but that has been impossible to obtain in cancer screening. Generally, we are forced to accept some kind of compromise between those two objectives. If not missing any cancer is our primary concern, then we'll be most interested in a test that is as sensitive as possible, knowing it will yield some false-positive results. If we care more about not subjecting healthy people to the rigors of further testing, we'll prefer a test that is adequately specific.

Here is a calculation, presented in a Viewpoint article in the *Journal of the American Medical Association*, that helps explain why screening commonly gives us misleading results: Assume we have a test that is 90 percent sensitive and 96 percent specific, which the authors point out is actually better than most screening tests. If it is used to screen for a type of cancer prevalent in 0.6 percent of the population, the test will turn up 40 false-positive results and find six people who actually have the condition for every 1,000 people screened. (The authors do not estimate how many cancers will be missed.)[3]

The false positives tell us we are getting data we can't accurately interpret. Perhaps the markers we are using—say a protein or an enzyme in the blood—sometimes indicate cancer and sometimes do not. Since we can't distinguish them, the warnings typically lead to action, but we may not be acting appropriately. A single screening test can trigger a cascade of potentially unnecessary medical events.

Even more surprising is that the six people whose cancers were detected in our hypothetical example may not gain an extra benefit from starting treatment early. Some cancerous changes in the cells never progress further, and others are so aggressive that finding them early doesn't change the prognosis. That's why the value of those tests may be exaggerated—we may not be saving as many lives as we thought.

"Most people who have their cancer detected early are not being helped," declares H. Gilbert Welch, MD, MPH, professor of medicine at the Dartmouth Institute for Health Policy and Clinical Practice, who has studied screening extensively. "Either they are being told they have cancer earlier than they would otherwise be told. Or worse, they are being treated unnecessarily for cancer that never would have bothered them."

"I've come to the conclusion that overdiagnosis is not the exception," agrees Barnett Kramer, MD, MPH, the director of the Division of Cancer Prevention at the NCI. "Any screening test can pick up tumors that do not need to be treated."

Yet patients who have had cancer detected by screening tend to think that they were lucky to catch it early. This is the "popularity paradox"[4]—screening finds a lot more cancer, more people become cancer survivors, and everyone assumes that screening saved their lives. That gives us a somewhat-elevated sense of the importance of such tests.

Beyond the possibility of providing misleading information, some screening tests also carry potential harms of their own. Mammography, for example, exposes a woman to small amounts of radiation over her lifetime, possibly raising her odds for cancer. In rare instances, colonoscopies result in a perforated colon. These are very small risks, but they cannot be ignored.

In addition, the follow-up required to evaluate a finding suspicious for cancer may also cause the patient harm, not to mention extreme stress. For example, if a chest x-ray or a lung CT scan looks abnormal—and that happens between 20 and 60 percent of the time among smokers—a lung biopsy will be necessary. To test the tissue, a physician will perform bronchoscopy, in which a scope is placed down the windpipe, and if a biopsy is taken, a needle is inserted through the airway. Either procedure can cause a partial collapse of the lung, bleeding, infection, and pain, although these occur infrequently. If a larger amount of tissue is needed for the biopsy, chest surgery may be necessary.

For all these reasons, there is a remarkable inconsistency in the screening guidelines of major professional organizations. More than 180 guidelines to detect cancer are posted on the National Guidelines

Clearinghouse, maintained by the federal Agency for Healthcare Research and Quality. While this centralized Web-based repository makes the information easy to access, the array of recommendations in one place also highlights the many contradictions in the field.

As Otis Brawley, MD, and his colleagues at the American Cancer Society (ACS) write in the *Journal of the American Medical Association,* "many cancer screening guidelines differ, even when purported to have been based on the same set of evidence. Those differences can cast doubt on the credibility of both the recommendations and the organizations that produced them."[5]

It's more evidence of the uncertainty in the field. If there were clear answers, expert opinion would not vary as much as it does.

THE PSA DEBATE

The prostate-specific antigen test may be the most controversial screening test in widespread use. Approved by the FDA in 1994, it detects blood levels of an enzyme made by the prostate, which can rise in the presence of prostate cancer. The appeal of early detection is obvious—an estimated 241,000 American men were diagnosed with prostate cancer in 2011, and almost 34,000 of them will die because of it.[6] Most men with prostate cancer are now being diagnosed through screening.[7]

The problem is that PSA levels fluctuate over time and can also be elevated in healthy men, especially those who have an enlarged prostate, a commonplace complaint of middle-age men known as benign prostatic hyperplasia, or who have an inflammatory condition called prostatitis. This is a clear example of a test that lacks adequate specificity.

Despite that, there is a textbook response to a high PSA score.

A biopsy is scheduled, and if the biopsy finds cancer cells, men are almost always advised to pursue further treatment, usually surgery, radiation, or hormonal therapy. This may be layering an unnecessary procedure on top of an unnecessary procedure, because prostate cancer can progress so slowly that some men do not actually require treatment.

PSA testing, explains the NCI's Dr. Barnett Kramer, "finds many silent tumors that never would have caused problems had they not been detected." Indeed, ongoing monitoring—known as watchful waiting—is appropriate in some cases, but relatively few physicians and patients feel confident enough to consider that option.

As a result, we are spending vast resources searching for prostate cancer in healthy people, and then treating some who may not need it. One study, co-authored by Richard J. Ablin, PhD, a researcher of immunology and pathology at the University of Arizona College of Medicine, suggests that we spend $5.2 million on screening, and the diagnostic and treatment measures that follow, to prevent a single prostate cancer death.[8]

The limitations of the PSA test are such that Ablin, who discovered the prostate-specific antigen, says it is "hardly more effective than a coin toss" and argues against its widespread use. In a *New York Times* op-ed piece, he writes, "Testing should absolutely not be deployed to screen the entire population of men over the age of 50. . . . I never dreamed that my discovery would lead to such a profit-driven public health disaster."[9]

What we need instead, says Dr. Kramer, is the ability "to distinguish those cancers that need to be treated from those that don't. We need to identify overdiagnosis at the molecular level so that we avoid it."

The US Preventive Services Task Force now agrees that our current prostate cancer screening approach is not supported by evidence. The task force, an independent panel of experts under congressional mandate, reviews available scientific evidence to provide guidelines for primary care providers and health systems. In an official recommendation statement issued in May 2012, the task force advised against having routine PSA screening at any age.[10] That is a firmer stance than it took in 2008, when it said that there was insufficient evidence to assess the benefits or harms of prostate cancer screening in men under 75.[11]

Still, many clinicians continue their routine use of PSA screenings. The American Urological Association still calls for PSA screening beginning at age 40, although it has said it will be developing new clinical guidelines.[12] Meanwhile, many doctors on the front lines continue to urge healthy men to have a PSA test.

"I've always been a believer that it's better to have information and to use that information to inform a man's decision," says Howard Scher, MD, chief of the genitourinary oncology service at Memorial Sloan-Kettering Cancer Center. "With more-judicious use of PSA testing, we can determine who needs surveillance; and if we see a change that suggests a cancer is becoming more aggressive, we can intervene."

The difference between the standardized recommendations and clinical practice reflects a tension that often exists between people who analyze data to generate what is known as "evidence-based guidelines" and people who actually treat patients. All their intentions are honorable, but the inconsistencies are very challenging for patients who must make decisions regarding screening on the basis of uncertain science.

At least there is some common ground here. Everyone agrees we desperately need better tests to distinguish between prostate cancers that need immediate treatment and those that can be safely moni-tored until there is a reliable signal telling us when the time for more medical intervention is truly at hand.

Concerns about Mammograms

Mammograms have also come under considerable criticism in recent years. Long thought to be a gold standard for breast cancer screening, the annual mammogram is a routine part of the lives of millions of American women. Most of them believe it plays a crucial role in finding breast cancer early and reducing deaths.

Here, too, the real value may be less than we once assumed.

The US Preventive Services Task Force states categorically that "there is convincing evidence" that screening reduces breast cancer deaths, with the greatest reductions for women ages 50 to 74.[13]

If that's the good news, the National Breast Cancer Coalition is skeptical of it. It points out that no mortality benefit was found in the two large, published clinical trials generally considered to be the most reliable on the topic. One of these enrolled 42,000 women, ages 45 to 69, and the other looked at almost 90,000 women, ages 40 to 59. The coalition says that results from five other key studies were generally weak, although cumulatively they did show a small reduction in risk.[14]

Other data also suggest that mammography has a small impact. One study found that 2,970 women must be screened once in order to save one life.[15] Another, published in *Archives of Internal Medicine*, found that 990 women with mammography-detected breast cancer, per 100,000 in the general population, would likely die of the disease over 20 years, compared with 1,240 women who did not have mammograms. That means that 250 women per 100,000 actually gained a benefit.[16]

Mammograms certainly find cancer earlier than we otherwise would have, but experts disagree about their impact on the course of the disease. According to an estimate published in the *Journal of the American Medical Association,* 3.5 of every 1,000 women in their 40s will die of breast cancer over the next 10 years if they are not screened. Screening will reduce that to about 3 in 1,000 deaths, according to this study. "For most women with cancer, screening generally does not change the ultimate outcome; the cancer usually is just as treatable or just as deadly regardless of screening," write the authors.[17]

Building on that kind of evidence, the task force revised its breast cancer screening recommendations. In 2002, it had said that all women should have a mammogram every year or two, starting at age 40.[18] Newer guidelines issued in 2009 recommended that women under 50 not be screened routinely, and that those 50 to 74 be screened only every two years. The task force also concluded that the evidence is inadequate to assess the benefits and harms of mammograms for those age 75 or beyond.[19]

Unfortunately, the recommendations are inconsistent across organizations. For example, the NCI still advises women age 40 or older to have mammograms every one or two years,[20] and the ACS and Susan G. Komen for the Cure still recommend annual mammograms for all women over 40.[21]

Many studies reinforce the benefits of regular mammography screening. In a 2009 Breast Cancer Symposium organized by the American Society of Clinical Oncology, researchers presented hospital data of nearly 7,000 women who had been diagnosed with invasive breast cancer. Eighty percent of them had been getting regular mammograms (defined as at least every two years) and 20 percent of them had not. Over a 13-year period, 461 of the women died from breast cancer: 75 percent of them were in the unscreened group. Based on their findings, the researchers estimated that screened women diagnosed with breast cancer will have a 13-year mortality rate of 5 percent compared to a 56 percent mortality rate for unscreened women.[22] The benefit of mammography in reducing the incidence of advanced breast cancer was reinforced in May 2012 in a review of 10 randomized controlled trials. This study emphasized the effectiveness of diagnosing breast cancer in its early stages, therefore reducing deaths due to breast cancer.[23]

Realizing this, many clinicians diverge even more sharply away from the task force recommendations. When I spoke with Julie Mitnick, MD, an associate professor of clinical radiology at New York University and the founder of Murray Hill Radiology and Mammography, a well-respected private radiology practice in New York, she suggested that some of the studies on which the task force conclusions were based might have been flawed. Dr. Mitnick also pointed out that the same data can be subject to different interpretations. Furthermore, she is concerned that raising doubts about mammograms may lead to reluctance on the part of insurers to reimburse for the service.

Jill Fishbane-Mayer, MD, an assistant attending professor of gynecology at Mt. Sinai Hospital in New York City, shares that view. "I ignore the US Preventive Services Task Force guidelines," she acknowledges. Dr. Fishbane-Mayer, who is herself a breast cancer survivor, urges her patients to have a baseline mammogram between the ages of 35 and 40, depending on the patient's family history, and then to have annual mammograms starting at 40. Her best clinical instinct tells her that scheduling mammograms less frequently for older women, and not at all for younger ones, as the task force recommends, is risky.

Dr. Mitnick and Dr. Fishbane-Mayer are both concerned about the same thing: that women will be diagnosed at a later stage of disease, require more aggressive treatment, and increase their risk of dying from breast cancer. Obviously, the task force is concerned about that, too, but sometimes the argument holds greater sway over clinicians who interact with patients on a daily basis, see the ravages of cancer close up, and are eager to prevent it.

It doesn't bring a lot of clarity to the situation, however. Without a consensus, everyone is left flailing here, with both patients and physicians making choices based primarily on clinical experience and personal preferences.

SMARTER WAYS TO USE OUR TOOLS

One of the best opportunities we have to use screening more wisely is to consider the individual circumstances of every patient. There's a significant difference between screening all healthy people for all cancers and targeting our tests more specifically to those who are most likely to develop a disease, or are most concerned about it. Family history, previous medical experiences, and smoking behavior are among the factors that can shift the risk-benefit equation for many kinds of tests.

In a recent *Annals of Internal Medicine* article, for example, researchers suggested that personalized, risk-based mammography screening might be the answer.[24] They concluded that extremely dense breasts or a first-degree relative with breast cancer doubled the risk of developing breast cancer in women, age 40 to 49. In that population, more frequent screening makes sense.

We also need to do a better job of getting more people screened with the tests about which we are completely confident. We are screening 83 percent of those in the target population for cervical cancer, while the federal government's Healthy People 2020 initiative has set a goal of screening just over 93 percent of them by 2020.[25]

The story of my friend Bridget is a deeply personal one that tells us what those statistics really mean. While she was in the midst of a brutal chemotherapy regimen after she had been diagnosed with cervical cancer, I asked her how she was doing. I still remember her words of anguish.

"I'm mad at *me*," she said.

She knew that if she had gone for regular gynecological checkups and Pap tests, her cancer would likely have been detected at its earliest stage, when it might have been still curable.

Even with the availability of an effective test, some 12,700 new cervical cancer cases occurred in 2011, and there were almost 4,300 deaths.[26]

Low screening rates for colon cancer are another concern. Colonoscopy not only finds cancer but also can be used to remove polyps before they become malignant; that's prevention in its optimal form. The test requires significant preparation, time, and patience, but with more than 141,000 cases of colon cancer and 49,000 deaths in 2011, it is a test that saves lives.[27]

Fewer than 59 percent of people who should be screened for colon cancer actually are, while the Healthy People's target rate for 2020 has been set just above 70 percent.[28] Current screening rates are considerably lower among a host of populations with more marginal access to the health care system, including people of color, less-educated populations, and those without insurance.

SCREENING FOR OTHER CANCERS

Along with improving the tests we currently have, we need effective screening for the many other cancers that lack good early-detection options. As we search for markers that we can measure and interpret accurately, we should avoid putting new tests in wide use until we really understand what they are telling us. Past experience should be our guide here—we don't advance the cause of prevention, or satisfy our passionate desire to intercept cancer, by offering tests that add more confusion to an already murky picture.

———

Much attention is being paid to how we can screen for two of the most lethal cancers—lung cancer and ovarian cancer—when they are in an early-enough stage to be curable.

Lung cancer is expected to cause more than 160,000 deaths in the United States in 2012, more than breast, colon, and prostate cancer combined. Because we lack good screening options for lung cancer, just 15 percent of cases are found early; when they are, half of those who are treated survive at least five years. If treatment does not begin until the cancer is more advanced, only 16 percent of people manage to live five years or more.[29] We haven't seen survival rates for lung cancer improve significantly since 1971. Survival rates for lung cancer rose a mere 2 percent between 1971 and 2010.[30]

Three techniques have been studied for their possible role in lung cancer screening: use of a low-dose CT scan, a chest x-ray, or sputum cytology, in which a microscope is used to look for abnormal cells in a mucus sample. The US Preventive Services Task Force said in 2004 that the evidence was insufficient to recommend any of these tools to people without symptoms.[31]

More hopeful news came in 2011, when the NCI's Prostate, Lung, Colon, and Ovary Screening Trial reported results from a study of nearly 54,000 current and former smokers, ages 55 to 74, with a history of heavy smoking. The trial compared screening with chest x-rays to screening via a low-dose spiral CT scan, a newer technology that provides high-resolution images as patients hold their breath. The study, reported in the *New England Journal of Medicine*, found that lung cancer deaths were reduced by an impressive 20 percent as a result of the CT scan.[32]

It's a promising finding, although we still need to learn more about the benefits and risks of CT scans. Right now, we don't know how useful the test is for a younger population or for light smokers, and we don't know how frequently smokers should be scanned. The test also had a high rate of false positives—about one in every four people had to undergo more testing to be sure no cancer was present. Radiation exposure is a further risk for this population.

Nonetheless, some advocates are already calling for new lung cancer screening guidelines based on the early findings. Carolyn R. Aldigé, founder of the Prevent Cancer Foundation in Alexandria, Virginia, which is dedicated to early cancer detection and prevention, hails the findings as the "biggest breakthrough in detecting early stage lung cancer."

For now, the ACS recommends that heavy smokers and ex-smokers, like the participants in the NCI's Prostate, Lung, Colon, and Ovary Screening Trial, discuss these screening options with their physicians.[33]

The need for an ovarian cancer screening test is also urgent. If it is caught at its earliest stage, when the cancer is still confined to the ovaries, women have a 94 percent chance of long-term survival.

More often, by the time a woman notices that she has symptoms and brings them to the attention of her doctor, the disease already may have spread.

Sadly, more than two-thirds of women aren't diagnosed until it has progressed to a stage III or IV cancer, when they have only an 18 to 45 percent chance of living another five years.[34] The fifth-leading cause of cancer deaths among women, ovarian cancer will be diagnosed in more than 22,000 women in 2012, and 15,500 women will die of the disease, according to the NCI.[35]

Ovarian cancer is particularly difficult to detect because the small, walnut-shaped ovaries are deep within a woman's pelvic cavity, where they can't readily be felt or seen on an x-ray or traditional ultrasound. The disease is known as "the silent killer."

Hope for early detection came with the symptom index, developed by Barbara Goff, MD, director of gynecologic oncology at the University of Washington School of Medicine in Seattle, and her colleagues.[36] By identifying a constellation of symptoms indicative of ovarian cancer—including frequent abdominal or pelvic pain, a strong or frequent need to urinate, abdominal bloating, and difficulty eating or a tendency to feel full quickly—the symptom index is designed to speed up the diagnosis of cancer. However, subsequent research has found that, in the real world, the symptom index has only a modest impact on the timing of the diagnosis.[37] In fact, the researchers suggest that, at best, using a symptom index would speed up a diagnosis by three months, and the impact of that extra time on survival is not known.

A screening test of real value would detect ovarian cancer before symptoms appear. One promising tool is a transvaginal ultrasound. Since 1987, the Ovarian Cancer Screening Research Program at the University of Kentucky's Markey Cancer Center has screened 37,000 women, found 500 lesions of concern, and determined with further testing that 60 of them were positive for cancer.[38] "We're looking for needles in haystacks, but we are finding them," says John R. van Nagell Jr., MD, the director of gynecologic oncology at the university, in a 2011 article dedicated to ovarian cancer in *Prevention*. As the data suggest, however, there are a lot of false positives and a lot of unnecessary surgeries to assess the lesions.

Another approach could involve measuring levels of CA-125, a protein in the blood that rises in some women with ovarian cancer. Researchers at MD Anderson Cancer Center in Dallas developed an algorithm that establishes normal, intermediate, and high-risk levels of CA-125 and tested it on more than 3,000 women over eight years. They retested women every three months if their CA-125 climbed into the intermediate range, and performed a transvaginal ultrasound if it reached the high-risk level.

Only a small percentage of women needed the quarterly blood tests, and even fewer needed the ultrasound. Eight women had follow-up surgery to search for ovarian cancer after a suspicious finding on a sonogram, and three of them were diagnosed with early-stage disease. The strength of this approach is that it establishes baseline CA-125 levels and a pattern over time, providing a measured approach that appears to limit false positives.[39]

A similar but much larger trial is under way in the United Kingdom, with results expected in 2014. The real value will come if that study shows the algorithm actually reduces the death rate of ovarian cancer. Unfortunately we've had an earlier disappointment on that score. The NCI's Prostate, Lung, Colon, and Ovary Screening Trial, which screened women with both the CA-125 and transvaginal ultrasound tests, did not show a mortality reduction.[40] For now, the ACS and the NCI both recommend against the routine use of either test for screening.[41]

In an ideal world, we will someday be able to offer sensitive and specific, life-extending screening for all cancers to all people. That remains a distant goal, but stands as one of the highest priorities in our drive toward prevention.

To get there, we will have to keep refining our current tests for detecting cancer and search more diligently for others that are more reliable. Until we can make uniform recommendations, doctors should be more candid with their patients about the limits of their current options.

Some will become informed consumers, reading up on the controversies and making personal screening choices on the basis of what matters most to them. Many will not, and that's reasonable, too. Not everyone should be expected to read the opinions on both sides of a medical question and cast their own ballot. Instead, they will follow the clinical judgment of their doctors, who will likely base their own recommendations on some combination of experience, clinical judgment, and habit.

That's the reality of where we are now, and it's not a satisfactory state of affairs. We simply don't have all the science we need to guide action. "Where is the universal blood test?" asks cancer pioneer James Holland, MD, a distinguished professor of neoplastic disease at the Mt. Sinai School of Medicine in New York.

To find a marker in the blood, or perhaps the urine, that is both sensitive and specific enough to detect cancer at its earliest stages remains one of our most pressing prevention objectives. The idea is to collect information from large populations quickly, inexpensively, and accurately, and to save lives in the process. Advancing toward that goal will demand more dedicated research efforts.

CHAPTER 4

CUT, POISON, AND BURN: A LOOK AT TODAY'S TREATMENT OPTIONS

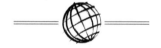

OR MOST OF THE 20TH CENTURY, WE HAVE USED three basic approaches to treat cancer: surgery, chemotherapy, and radiation. With experimentation and practice, we have become better able to target all of them more precisely at cancer cells, and we have learned how to counteract some of their side effects. Our surgical techniques have grown more refined, our chemical arsenal has become larger, and our radiation beams take more exacting aim.

Yet, our results remain entirely inadequate. Each approach has short-term and long-term risks and too often allows cancer to return. In crude fashion, we are still trying to cut, poison, and burn our way through cancer. "My treatment imperils my health," declares actor Cynthia Nixon in a powerful Broadway revival of *Wit,* Margaret Edson's signature play about a woman with advanced ovarian cancer.

Chemotherapy can be especially grueling, with many patients receiving one drug after another. "Usually the first treatment regimen works and then it stops working after a certain point," says Dr. Nicholas Vogelzang of the American Society of Clinical Oncology. "For certain cancers you can go on indefinitely treating some patients, provided they don't have organ failure. I have one patient who has had 13 different treatments for metastatic prostate cancer. I have a kidney patient who is on program number 10. I saw a woman with ovarian cancer the other day who had 11."

That these patients remain alive, albeit seriously ill, is certainly good news. Many others haven't been so lucky. If we need a persuasive argument for shifting our focus to prevention, surely we can find it in the toxic, invasive, and sometimes disfiguring alternatives that we currently offer. Yet the best scientific minds in the pharmaceutical industry, the research establishment, and the medical profession remain focused on treatment.

Although I strongly believe that our priorities are misplaced, I don't want to diminish the cancer success stories we do have. After surgery and radiation, early breast cancer may never return. Some skin moles can simply be removed and the cancer they contain is gone. Hodgkin's disease, acute lymphatic leukemia, and testicular cancer can truly be cured with chemotherapy.

For most cancer patients, cancer treatment is an arduous and debilitating experience. Gregg experienced many of cancer's challenges firsthand. His ordeal began at age 59 when a routine x-ray showed a spot on the lower lobe of his left lung. Gregg, a smoker since early adulthood, was diagnosed with non-small cell lung cancer, the most common form of the disease.

The tumor was removed during surgery, and then Gregg endured six months of chemotherapy. When the veins in his arms became too "beat up" to tolerate more needles, doctors inserted a port into a neck vein to continue treatment.

All too soon, a follow-up CAT scan detected another tumor, this time in the upper portion of Gregg's right lung, and he underwent eight weeks of radiation therapy. To reach the tumor's awkward location, the radiologist had to shoot radiation through his esophagus. Gregg was warned that his throat would likely be too sore to eat or drink normally for some time to come and that he would need intravenous nutrition. He was lucky in that he actually put on weight during treatment. "By the end of the treatment, I had gained 30 pounds and was eating and drinking with as much gusto as ever," he says. That gave everyone some hope.

For a year, Gregg was considered to be in remission, with no obvious signs of cancer. Then, new growths were detected in various areas of the lungs, and a tumor was found in one of his adrenal glands. That indicated metastatic disease, and Gregg's prognosis was dismal—he had stage IV lung cancer. Just 1 percent of people with non-small cell lung cancer live five more years after the diagnosis.[1]

Defying all predictions, Gregg's cancer seemed to have been slowed by a steady procession of chemotherapy drugs, although he suffered greatly in exchange for those extra years of life. One drug caused an irregular heartbeat, another an abnormally rapid one. He had a tiny stroke behind his right eye. A chemotherapy agent his doctors tried in 2007 suppressed his bone marrow so severely that his white blood cell count plunged, putting him at risk for a life-threatening infection. To counteract that danger, he took yet another medication, this one designed to stimulate the growth of white blood cells.

After a genetic mutation was identified in one of his tumors, oncologists recommended a two-drug combination that gave him an acutely uncomfortable rash. He was advised to avoid the sun to control the rash, and that led to a significant vitamin D deficiency.

When a PET scan in 2010 showed two more cancerous nodules in his left lung, Gregg agreed to a high-dose radiation treatment delivered through the CyberKnife Robotic Radiosurgery System. Gregg found that treatment harrowing and began taking anti-anxiety medication prior to each of the 45-minute sessions, which are scheduled almost daily for two weeks.

Although he was grateful to survive until 2012, far beyond what was expected, Gregg's quality of life was significantly diminished. Gregg was engaged in a constant battle with cancer. "Cancer demands a good long fight," he said. "I would tell other cancer patients, 'Get ready for the fight of your life. Fight it with humor, and ignore, ignore, ignore the side effects as much as you can. Be as mean to your cancer as you possibly can. You can't be kind and gentle with cancer.'"

Given the limited tools available to doctors today, that's the right attitude for patients to have. However, as healers, we physicians would like to be much more effective. Surely, damaging the health of those who turn to us for help should not be the best we can do.

Let's take a brief look at the treatment options you could expect to hear about if you were diagnosed with cancer tomorrow. I can think of no more powerful way to communicate the message that our entire approach to cancer needs to be overhauled.

CUTTING: THE SURGICAL OPTION

Primitive forms of surgery have been in use for centuries, long before the era of anesthesia and antibiotics. Tumors in the arms and legs were once removed by amputation. A radical mastectomy, which removes not only the entire breast but the underlying chest muscles as well, used to be standard treatment for women with breast cancer, even in its earliest stages. Until the advent of scanning tools such as ultrasounds, MRIs, and PET scans in the latter part of the 20th century, we often subjected patients to exploratory surgery, with surgeons cutting into the body just to take a look around.

So, while surgery remains a routine part of cancer treatment, we certainly have made progress in how and when we cut into patients. If we are reasonably sure that a tumor has not spread beyond the organ in which it was first identified, surgery sometimes holds the promise of a full cure, with no further treatment necessary. More often, surgery is only a first step, to be followed by radiation or chemotherapy, or both. An alternative approach in some circumstances is to first treat cancer with radiation or chemotherapy, sometimes in the hopes of reducing the size of the tumor to allow for less extensive surgery.

Depending on the nature, extent, and aggressiveness of the cancer cells, a surgeon may advise removing a cancerous organ entirely or cutting out only the tumor, leaving most or part of the organ intact. Where a partial excision is feasible, the goal is to obtain what we call a clear margin around the cancerous area—that is, a border of healthy tissue that contains no evidence of cancer cells. A clear margin reduces the risk that the cancer will recur, but there is no strict agreement on how large it should be, leaving surgeons to make decisions based on their professional judgment.[2]

Once the tissue is removed, a pathologist stains a tissue specimen with a special ink that makes it possible to distinguish cancerous cells from normal ones. If a pathology report later indicates that cancer cells are present within the tissue surrounding the visible tumor, or if a doctor feels that a larger margin area is needed, a patient will sometimes be advised to return for a second operation.

Unfortunately, we see this happening too often in the treatment of breast cancer. Asking patients to return to the operating table so that further cuts can be made into their breast tissue has "significant physical, psychological and financial effects," researchers reported in the *Journal of the American Medical Association*, with a degree of understatement.[3] While such surgeries may sometimes be necessary, the study revealed significant inconsistencies, across surgeons and medical institutions, in the frequency with which women are scheduled for a second surgical operation. That raises questions about whether doctors are basing their recommendations for follow-up surgery—and the trauma that inevitably accompanies it—on solid evidence.

As with screening, this is another medical practice that seems to be based more on physician habits than on scientific evidence. Cancer surgery can be approached in numerous ways, and where possible, patient preferences should be considered in the choice. Surgeons may differ in how much tissue they want to take, where they cut into the body to gain access to the tumor, and whether they think newer forms of surgery, such as robotics or laparoscopic procedures, are appropriate. Where the decisions affect quality of life in either the short or long term, patients should get detailed, comprehensible information about the pros and cons of various options. Unfortunately, few consistent guidelines are in place to ensure that they do.

Breast cancer again offers a good example. For many years, women were told that their entire breast had to be removed once cancer was found. Yet, study after study, including one that followed more than 2,000 women for 20 years, has shown that a lumpectomy, in which only the tumor and a clear margin around it are cut out, is just as effective when combined with radiation.[4]

Despite the evidence, some women are never even told by their doctors that a lumpectomy may be appropriate. It's not for everybody, and there can be good reasons to opt for more extensive surgery, but there is almost never a justification for not presenting all the risks and benefits of both approaches. The real surgical problem, as an editorial in the *New England Journal of Medicine* pointed out, is not that cancer could recur locally if the breast is preserved, but that "many women today are not offered the option of breast-conserving therapy."[5]

That attitude may be due in part "to the American tendency to think that more is always better in virtually any situation," wrote Susan Love, MD, a pioneering advocate of multidisciplinary breast care for women and the author of the "bible" on the topic, *Dr.*

Susan Love's Breast Book.[6] "If it hurts more or it's a bigger operation, it must be the best."

Compelling data tell us that for breast cancer, that's wrong, and a less aggressive, less debilitating approach to surgery can be appropriate for many women. As the *New England Journal* editorial proclaimed, "It is time to declare the case against breast-conserving therapy closed and focus our efforts on new strategies for the prevention and cure of breast cancer."[7]

———

Steve Jobs, the legendary founder of Apple, died of pancreatic cancer in 2011, eight years after he was diagnosed. With five-year survival rates for pancreatic cancer averaging just about 6 percent, media across the country ran long articles about how he had beaten the odds. In *Scientific American,* Katherine Harmon pointed out that wasn't actually quite true: The Apple CEO had a rare form of the disease known as a pancreatic neuroendocrine tumor, which has a much longer survival time.[8]

Still, the disease took his life at the age of 56. As head of one of the world's most profitable companies, Jobs could have had access to any treatment available, anywhere in the world. Unfortunately, he simply didn't have a lot of good options, and he ran out of time. Neither power nor wealth could make the modified Whipple procedure he underwent any less harrowing.

One of the most invasive of all cancer surgeries, the Whipple procedure involves removing parts of the pancreas, bile duct, and small intestine, as well as the gallbladder, nearby lymph nodes, and sometimes parts of the stomach. Even in the most capable surgical hands, the procedure carries a high risk of postoperative complications, including infection, bleeding, and leakage from the new connections that are made between the tissues and organs that remain in the body.

Admittedly, the Whipple procedure is a lot safer than it once was. In the 1970s, as many as 25 percent of the patients who had the surgery died as a result of it. Today, at major medical centers that have a lot of experience performing the Whipple procedure, that figure has fallen to less than 5 percent. Still, life is never quite the same for someone who has had the procedure, which increases the likelihood of developing diabetes, often makes digesting food difficult, and can cause significant diarrhea. With a 20 percent chance of a cure, some people decide those risks are worth taking even though the long-term odds of beating the cancer are poor. I find myself wondering, as I so often do, whether this is really the best we can offer.

Sometimes, surgery isn't an option. Tumors may be inoperable because they are located in an area that's almost impossible to reach, or a patient may not be strong enough to withstand surgery. If cancer has spread far enough, doctors may conclude that an operation will only weaken a patient's stamina without offering a meaningful benefit.

Even if someone does undergo surgery, there is no way to be sure it has been successful. Although every cancer patient yearns to hear the words "we got it all," cancer has the capacity to lurk in nearby tissues, even where a clear margin seems to have been obtained, or to spread undetected through the blood or lymph nodes. For all these reasons, chemotherapy and other therapies are usually recommended as a standard part of contemporary cancer care.

POISONS: THE LIMITS OF ANTICANCER DRUGS

Pharmaceuticals are a mainstay of treatment. Collectively called "systemic therapy," these include three major groups: chemotherapy, targeted therapy, and hormonal therapy. In various combinations, these drugs may be used on their own or teamed with surgery and radiation to attack cancer cells. Administered prior to surgery or radiation, they are called neoadjuvant therapy; the same drugs administered afterward are called adjuvant therapy.

Physicians sometimes avoid the technical language and simply call them "poison"—what we want the drugs to do is kill cancer cells. Unfortunately, they can kill normal, healthy cells as well. As actor Anna Deavere Smith says in her powerful one-woman show *Let Me Down Easy,* "chemotherapy is like taking a stick and beating a dog to get rid of fleas."

"Poison" is also an apt term because the first chemotherapeutic agent to play a role in medicine was closely related to mustard gas, an agent of chemical warfare in World Wars I and II. After observing that soldiers who had been exposed to mustard gas had depleted cells in their bone marrow and lymph nodes, scientists at Yale University began studying the potential value of mustard compounds in cancer treatment.

In one experiment, they transplanted a tumor into the lymph tissue of mice and found that nitrogen mustard caused it to regress. The researchers delayed publishing their results until 1946, when the war's end lifted the veil of secrecy over the use of toxic chemicals. Once they did reveal their findings, nitrogen mustard came into widespread use to treat lymphomas, the cancers of the lymphoid tissue.

Soon enough, the regression of lymphoma tumors proved to be incomplete and short-lived, and hope was replaced by disappointment. That seems to have set a pattern that continues to this day, with one promising therapy after another swept up in a fever of excitement, only to eventually be discarded once we become aware of its limitations.

Still, the initial success with nitrogen mustard suggested that we might eventually be able to cure cancer with drugs, and the search was on for others. Pushed by the relentless Mary Lasker, Congress gave $5 million to the National Cancer Institute (NCI) to establish the Cancer Chemotherapy National Service Center, which was up and running by 1955. The initiative, since renamed the Developmental Therapeutics Program, continues to this day.

Its creation helped define the treatment-oriented cancer agenda that still dominates research. "Without question it changed the face of cancer drug development in the world," said Vincent DeVita Jr. and Edward Chu in their fascinating history of cancer chemotherapy, published in *Cancer Research*. "It gave birth to the multibillion-dollar cancer pharmaceutical industry."[9]

Also, without question, fighting cancer remains highly profitable. The drug companies have all the incentive to keep their research focused on developing powerful therapies, rather than on eliminating cancer altogether. Billions of dollars in revenue are at stake.

Should we really dedicate ourselves to changing behavior, eliminating environmental carcinogens, or finding low-cost supplements that reduce cancer risks, the drug industry is likely to feel a blow to its bottom line. Prevention may yet offer some revenue-generating opportunities—for example, in the area of vaccine development—but in all probability, profits will decline.

＿＿＿

There are various classes of chemotherapy drugs, but they all share the goal of killing rapidly dividing cells.

Chemotherapy is administered intravenously or through a combination of intravenous drip and pills, on a schedule that depends on the type of drug and the nature of the cancer. It might be daily, every other day, once a week, or even once every four or six weeks. To increase the effectiveness of chemotherapy and to minimize the capacity of cancer cells to develop resistance, oncologists may administer more than one drug at a time or use different treatments in sequence. If a cancer returns after treatment—in other words, when "first-line" therapy stops being effective—there is typically more in the tool chest to offer. Even if second-line and third-line therapies fail, we can usually find something new, but rarely is it something that will work well for very long.

The toxic effects of chemotherapy are not limited to cancer cells. Every drug has its own package of debilitating and sometimes-bizarre side effects. Some of these occur during treatment and immediately afterward; some occur five or more years later. The most familiar are fatigue, lack of appetite, nausea, diarrhea or constipation, and hair loss. Chemotherapy can also cause neuropathy, or damage to the nerves, leading to pain and numbness in the hands and feet. Other complaints include sharp pain, muscle aches, the feeling of being pricked by pins and needles, burns, a sore or dry mouth, and rashes that can be almost intolerably itchy. In young women, chemotherapy may accelerate the onset of menopause, with its accompanying hot flashes and mood swings.

The risk of infection is particularly acute because treatment can lower a person's white blood cell count, a condition known as neutropenia. Sepsis, a potentially fatal blood infection, can occasionally result. Drugs can also lower the red blood cell count, leaving a patient feeling short of breath or anemic, or reduce platelet counts, causing bleeding that won't stop.

Some patients develop a condition that has been dubbed "chemo brain," a mental cloudiness with symptoms that include forgetfulness, difficulty concentrating, and slower mental functioning. While this has generally been thought to be a short-term problem, a number of studies have reported changes in cognition five years after chemotherapy. In a particularly alarming study published in the *Journal of Clinical Oncology,* researchers suggested that the effects can endure even longer than that. They conducted a series of tests on women treated with a three-drug chemotherapy regimen 20 years earlier and found their performance to be "significantly worse" than that of a healthy comparison group.[10]

Other effects also can develop long after treatment. The specific impact depends on the type of cancer and the types of drugs used to treat it, but higher-dose therapies administered for longer periods of time generally carry the greatest risks. According to the American Society of Clinical Oncology, late effects can strike just about anywhere in the body—including the heart, lungs, brain and spinal cord, bones and joints, and endocrine and digestive systems. Even dental and vision problems can occur.

When the drug doxorubicin (Adriamycin), for example, is used to treat childhood leukemia, the survivors may have diminished heart function when they reach adulthood.[11] Adults treated with doxorubicin for bladder, breast, lung, stomach, or ovarian cancer can also experience heart damage years after treatment. Five percent of patients who took a relatively low cumulative dose (400 mg/m²) had congestive heart failure, and as the dose rose, so did the risk. One-quarter of the patients using doxorubicin at a dose of 550 mg/m² experienced heart failure.[12]

Folfirinox, a four-drug chemotherapy regimen to treat metastatic pancreatic cancer, can extend life about four months longer than the more commonly used single agent, gemcitabine. Its powerful side effects—including neuropathy, gastrointestinal complaints, and severe neutropenia, which increases the risk for infections that can lead to sepsis—can greatly diminish the quality of life during those final months.[13]

Then there are the secondary cancers—cancers of a different type than the one originally diagnosed—that these treatments can predispose patients to. Leukemia is the most common type of cancer to develop following chemotherapy. Typically, a patient will develop myelodysplastic syndrome, a condition affecting bone marrow, which can then turn into acute myelogenous leukemia. Among the widely used chemotherapies most associated with leukemia are a class of drugs called alkylating agents, as well as cisplatin and topoisomerase II inhibitors.[14]

Even drugs used to treat the side effects of chemotherapy have been linked to secondary cancers. For example, patients who need medication to raise their white blood cell counts may be injected with granulocyte colony stimulating factor (G-CSF), a substance normally found in the blood. Researchers observed that this doubled the risk of developing either myelodysplastic syndrome or acute myelogenous leukemia.[15]

When it comes to chemotherapy, no patient emerges unscathed, and the benefits may not last. If cancer cells become resistant to chemotherapy, as often happens over time, they begin to multiply again. The question for patients is always whether the gain in longevity will ultimately outweigh the brutality of the treatment.

A newer kind of poison is targeted therapy, designed to interfere with specific molecules within cancer cells. Targeted therapy evolved from the federal government's Special Virus Cancer Program, which was established in 1964 to identify viruses associated with cancer. When that strategy stalled, it was transformed into the Program of Molecular Biology, which has been immensely important in identifying oncogenes, suppressor oncogenes, and signaling pathways. The program facilitated the development of new targeted therapies and helped to produce technology that supported the sequencing of the human genome.[16]

Used alone or in combination with other drugs, targeted therapies attack cancer cells in a variety of ways. Some are designed to block the signals that tell cancer cells to keep dividing, others activate the immune system to destroy those cells, and still others send toxic substances into the cells or induce the programmed cell death known as apoptosis.

The FDA has approved a number of targeted therapies, and many others are in trials. By taking more direct aim at molecular targets, the hope is that these therapies will be more effective in killing cancer cells while doing less harm to healthy ones. That seems a distant promise, because for now, most of the drugs are prohibitively expensive, cause serious side effects, and typically extend life only a few weeks or months longer than standard treatments would.

Targeted cancer therapies include drugs and other substances that affect cell growth and the spread of cancer cells, and also influence the process by which cancer cells die. Among these targeted therapies are the monoclonal antibodies, which bind to cancer cells. A glimpse at four monoclonal antibodies helps to illustrate the limitations of the options we have available.

One of the best known is trastuzumab (Herceptin), which appears to interfere with certain growth-promoting signals of cancer cells. Teamed with other anticancer drugs, it is used to treat HER-2 positive breast cancer, as well as metastatic stomach cancer. Patients who use Herceptin may develop infections, diarrhea, and a low white blood cell count that is accompanied by fever. The drug also carries the risk of serious heart and lung problems.

Bevacizumab (Avastin) generated tremendous excitement when it came on the market—until its marginal benefits and troubling side effects tamped down expectations. The drug can cause high blood pressure, gastrointestinal perforation, stroke, heart attack, and bleeding that can be fatal. When it is added to other cancer regimens, the risk that those regimens will cause a fatal reaction increases significantly.[17]

Then there is ipilimumab (Yervoy), used to fight metastatic melanoma. Its manufacturer is required to provide the following safety information: "Can cause serious side effects in many parts of your body which can lead to death. These serious side effects may include inflammation of the intestines (colitis) that can cause tears or holes (perforation) in the intestines; inflammation of the liver (hepatitis) that can lead to liver failure; inflammation of the skin that can lead to severe skin reaction (toxic epidermal necrolysis); inflammation of the nerves that can lead to paralysis; inflammation of hormone-producing glands (especially the pituitary, adrenal, and thyroid glands) that may affect how these glands work; and inflammation of the eyes."[18]

The side effects of imatinib mesylate (Gleevec), which blocks the production of abnormal proteins thought to play a role in certain cancers, range from the fairly manageable (diarrhea, indigestion) to the potentially serious (shortness of breath; swelling of the extremities; fast, irregular, or pounding heartbeat; fainting; coughing up pink or bloody mucus; and jaundice).[19] Unlike the other monoclonal antibodies, however, imatinib really did transform one cancer, chronic myeloid leukemia (CML), into a manageable disease, giving patients a normal life expectancy.[20] Granted, CML may be a special case, because it involves a single molecular abnormality rather than the multiple abnormalities associated with most cancers.

Nevertheless, imatinib can be considered a success story. If only we had more of those.

———

Finally, we have the hormonal therapies, which are used to treat the hormone-fueled cancers of the breast, uterus, and prostate. These work by interfering with the hormones that promote cell growth or by stopping the body from making those hormones. The hormonal therapies target estrogen, a female sex hormone, and androgen, a male sex hormone.

One class of drugs, known as selective estrogen receptor modifiers, acts against estrogen in some tissues but behaves like estrogen in others. The anti-estrogen effects help block the hormonal stimulation of cancer cells in breast tissue. At the same time, the estrogenic properties of those same drugs increase the risk of uterine cancer and the possibility of major blood clots.

In 1999, researchers at the National Surgical Adjuvant Breast and Bowel Project, which has been conducting NCI–funded clinical trials for more than 50 years, launched the Study of Tamoxifen and Raloxifene (STAR) trial. One of the largest studies ever conducted to find ways to prevent invasive breast cancer, it assessed the value of two selective estrogen receptor modifiers: tamoxifen (Nolvadex) and raloxifene (Evista). Almost 20,000 high-risk postmenopausal women enrolled at more than 500 sites across the United States and Canada to compare the safety and effectiveness of the two drugs. In 2006, researchers demonstrated that both had cut the likelihood of developing invasive disease in half, and that raloxifene carried lower risks of uterine cancer and blood clots.[21]

Oncologists were understandably thrilled to have a proven prevention tool for women, although the risks of significant side effects, including uterine cancer and blood clots, remain a concern. Nonetheless, it is an important step in the right direction, and confirms that pharmaceutical research must be part of creating a world without cancer. It is not a magic pill, however—given the risk-benefit equation—and the US Preventive Services Task Force recommends against the routine use of tamoxifen or raloxifene to prevent breast cancer in postmenopausal women who are only at average risk for the disease.

Aromatase inhibitors are newer hormonal therapies that lower estrogen levels in the body by interfering with a key enzyme that would otherwise convert certain hormones into estrogen. FDA-approved aromatase inhibitors include anastrozole (Arimidex), exemestane (Aromasin), and letrozole (Femara). Exemestane is used to treat advanced breast cancer and to prevent recurrent breast cancer in postmenopausal women who have already been treated with tamoxifen and is being studied for its possible role in preventing cancer in high-risk women. While aromatase inhibitors apparently do not raise the risk of uterine cancer and are less likely to cause blood clots than tamoxifen, several studies indicate that the longer a woman uses them, the greater her chance of developing heart disease and osteoporosis.[22]

For men, a variety of androgen-deprivation drugs are available to reduce male hormones or to block the hormonal action that can stimulate the growth of prostate cancer. Standard treatment for prostate cancer that has spread beyond the prostate gland or returned after surgery or radiation, these drugs are often accompanied by a panoply of side effects, including impaired sexual function, weakened bones, hot flashes, diarrhea, vomiting, and itchiness. An alarming new study has also suggested that by destroying androgen-dependent cancer cells, these drugs may clear a path that allows neuroendocrine tumors to flourish.[23]

BURN: RADIATION THERAPY

The life of that childhood role model of mine, Marie Curie, suggests both the good and the bad of radiation as a clinical tool. Born in 1867, Madame Curie was a bold pioneer in the field of radioactivity. She recognized the potential of her work in medicine and set the stage for some of the immense breakthroughs that followed in the 20th century. Yet her death at the age of 67 from leukemia came almost surely because of her prolonged exposure to radiation.

And so it goes with radiation therapy as a cancer treatment. High-energy radiation, such as x-rays, gamma rays, and charged particles, is designed to kill cancer cells or damage their DNA in a way that keeps them from dividing. The goal may be to destroy a tumor; to shrink the tumor prior to surgery, allowing for a less-invasive procedure; or to use radiation after surgery to reach any cancer cells inadvertently left behind. In some circumstances, radiation may also be used to relieve pain, such as by shrinking a tumor exerting pressure on the spine.

The dose and schedule will vary, but in the United States about half of all patients diagnosed with cancer will be advised to have radiation therapy, before, during, or after surgery. Although we have gotten much better at aiming radiation directly at a tumor, we can't target it with the precision necessary to burn only cancer cells and leave healthy ones intact. That means that this therapy, too, is damaging.

Depending on the cancer and other variables, radiation can be administered in one of three ways: from outside the body, from within the body, or systemically.

External-beam therapy delivers radiation from a machine called a linear accelerator. Because the radiation is delivered from a distance, there is a risk that the beam can scatter and affect other parts of the body, although newer techniques are designed to prevent that. One popular approach is 3-D conformal radiation therapy, which uses radiation beams shaped to match the tumor so that a lower dose can be aimed more accurately. Intensity-modulated therapy adds further precision by varying the dose for different areas of the tumor and surrounding tissue. There are also external-beam techniques that use imaging scans for greater accuracy.

With internal radiation, also known as brachytherapy, radioactive isotopes sealed in tiny seedlike pellets are implanted in the body, near the cancer cells they are designed to damage. Best known as a treatment for prostate cancer, brachytherapy can be used for many other types of cancer as well. When it is administered at low doses, internal radiation typically remains in the body for days or weeks, and then the seeds are removed. High-dose internal radiation may be used repeatedly, but only for a few minutes at a time. Another technique involves permanent implants with a dose of radiation that gradually diminishes over time. In theory, internal radiation can provide higher-dose radiation with less damage to healthy cells.

Another tool is systemic radiation, which uses radioactive tracers that are injected or swallowed. Typically, these are bound to a drug designed to guide the radioactive substance to tumor cells.

Determining the value of radiation, as with surgery and chemotherapy, is a matter of weighing the benefits and the risks likely to be involved. Radiation appears to play an important role in eliminating some cancers. A 2011 *Lancet* study found that the risk of breast cancer recurrence was cut in half for patients who had radiation following a lumpectomy, compared with those who only had surgery.[24] Radiation therapy can also be a cure for prostate cancer confined to the prostate gland—although we don't have good evidence on which kind of radiation is most effective, or whether it is superior to surgery or even to no treatment at all.[25]

Research indicates that advising patients to undergo radiation is not always appropriate. Its routine use among elderly patients following surgery for stage III non-small cell lung cancer does not have a scientific basis, according to a team led by a Mt. Sinai School of Medicine researcher in New York. In an article published in *Cancer*, the team concluded that radiation did not increase survival time.[26]

Another study found that women treated with brachytherapy were twice as likely to have a mastectomy within five years—a likely indication that new signs of cancer had been found—compared with women treated with external-beam radiation.[27]

The side effects of any kind of radiation depend largely on the area of the body being treated and the intensity of the dose, as well as on the patient's overall health. Most patients complain of fatigue, which tends to intensify over the course of treatment. Acute side effects caused by radiation can also include skin irritation, damage to the salivary glands, urinary problems (if the abdominal area has been treated), and sometimes nausea. While many of these eventually disappear, some can linger for a long time or become permanent.

Months or even years after radiation, chronic side effects can surface. With radiation, as with chemotherapy, the list of potential problems is lengthy and alarming; it includes loss of motion in the joints, lymphedema (a swelling in the arms or legs), infertility, dental or mouth problems, and memory loss.

Most troubling is the possibility that other cancers will emerge, often near the original cancer site, long after receiving radiation therapy. Developing bodies are most sensitive to its effects, with more-advanced disease and treatment at younger ages associated with the greatest dangers. One study showed that children who survived cancer were 15 times more likely to die of a subsequent cancer later in life.[28]

Recently, researchers at Memorial Sloan-Kettering Cancer Center reported that 24 percent of childhood cancer survivors and 30 percent of women who received high-dose radiation therapy to the chest area to treat childhood Hodgkin's lymphoma developed breast cancer by the time they were 50 years old. These findings have significant implications for women with a history of radiation therapy in childhood, necessitating vigilant surveillance for breast cancer. By comparison, the average risk of breast cancer by age 50 is about 4 percent for most women and about 31 percent for carriers of a BRCA1 mutation.[29]

We also know that women who have had radiation therapy in

one breast before the age of 45 have a greater chance of developing a cancer in the other breast 10 years after treatment.

While radiation treatments have changed since these long-term follow-up studies, we don't yet know how this will ultimately affect the risk of developing a second cancer.

Though the young are most vulnerable, secondary cancers can develop as a result of radiation at any age. Breast cancer radiation seems to carry a particularly higher risk, and may be associated with subsequent lung cancer, as well as cancers of the blood vessels, bone, and connective tissues. The American Cancer Society says these cancers generally do not occur for 10 years after radiation therapy, but some of the risks remain elevated even 30 years later.

Women who have received radiation for ovarian cancer may be more likely to develop cancers of connective tissues, the bladder, and the pancreas, while radiation for cervical cancer raises the risk of cancers of the colon, rectum, small intestine, uterus, ovary, kidney, soft tissue, and stomach.

Men treated with radiation for prostate cancer subsequently have a higher risk of cancers of the bladder, colon, and rectum, compared with men who had surgery. Those same risks, as well as others, are evident after radiation for testicular cancer.

Radiation exposure is also associated with leukemia (including acute myelogenous, chronic myelogenous, and acute lymphoblastic leukemias). The risk depends on how much radiation was administered over what period of time, and the nature and level of the bone marrow's exposure to the radiation. The peak risk for developing leukemia usually occurs five to nine years after radiation exposure, and then declines slowly over time.

What all this tells us is that, once again, we have a treatment that initially works well for some people some of the time but in the long run fails to deliver a cure and carries significant side effects.

If the cut, poison, and burn regimens we currently offer worked better, the mix of side effects could more easily be justified by the result. However, combine the uncertain advantages with the horrors of treatment and it is not surprising that some people opt out somewhere along the way. Breast cancer patient Carole Baggerly, who founded Grassroots Health to address the worldwide problem of vitamin D deficiency, rejected her final round of paclitaxel because of the severe nerve pain it was causing. "I couldn't even walk," she recalls. "I refused to take any more of it."

She was also alarmed by the effect of her radiation treatment. Initially hesitant, she decided to accept her oncologist's reassurance that the side effects would be minimal, only to develop a red, oozing burn on her chest and more redness on her back. "It was extremely painful," she recalls. "The fact that the redness went through to my back was proof that the x-rays had scattered."

The fact that we have made so little progress after a century of using the same basic techniques surely suggests that we aren't taking the right approach. The problem? "Even one cancer cell can lead to death," says James Holland, MD, a distinguished professor of neoplastic diseases at Mt. Sinai School of Medicine in New York City. "Relapse is always a possibility until we can guarantee that there are no cancer cells in the body."

When death can come from a single cell that successfully eludes our most brutal attempts to cut, poison, and burn it, the sword of Damocles hangs over every patient's head.

CHAPTER 5

WHAT THE MARKET WILL BEAR

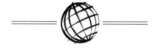

THE BRUTALITY OF CURRENT CANCER TREAT-
ment comes at a very high price. Our attempt to keep cancer at bay has become incredibly expensive, with drugs
playing a leading role in pushing up costs.

If we calculate only the direct costs of medical care, including
pharmaceuticals and the fees of physicians, hospitals, and other providers, we see a rise of about 75 percent from 1995 to 2004. By
2004, diagnostic tests and treatment cost about $70 billion, or about
5 percent of the nation's total spending on medical treatment.[1]

By 2010, that figure had reached an estimated $125 billion, and
there's no end in sight. Total direct costs of cancer care are estimated to reach $158 billion by 2020, according to research pub-

lished in the *Journal of the National Cancer Institute*.[2] That figure could be even higher, since it is adjusted only for the rising costs associated with the aging and growth of the US population. If the incidence of cancer increases, if drugs and other prices rise even further, or if we are able to keep people alive longer with more treatment, it could easily be more than $200 billion.

Factor lost productivity as a result of illness or early death into the equation and the numbers become truly stratospheric. With those indirect costs of cancer included, the total climbed to almost $210 billion in 2005[3] and reached nearly $264 billion in 2010.[4]

However we do the math, the numbers tell us one consistent thing: The cost of cancer to individuals and to society has risen inexorably over the past two decades. Cancer drugs alone are a huge component of this.

"The spiraling cost of cancer therapies has no villain," wrote Tito Fojo, MD, PhD, of the National Cancer Institute (NCI), and his colleagues. "Forces contributing to it include the pharmaceutical industry, academicians, professional societies, and practicing oncologists. These have collided with patients with cancer, navigating desperately in a perfect storm."[5]

I would suggest a slightly different perspective. No single villain, perhaps, but plenty of shared responsibility for a cancer culture that bears an unsustainable cost.

Promoting Cancer Drugs

With 887 cancer medicines and vaccines either in clinical trials or under review by the FDA as of 2011, drug costs will almost certainly continue to soar. "We don't have any cancer products in our pipeline that will be priced at less than $300,000" per quality-adjusted year of life, one pharmaceutical executive told Scott Ramsey, MD, PhD, director of Cancer Outcomes Research at the Fred Hutchinson Cancer Research Center in Seattle. Dr. Ramsey reported that conversation in the *Journal of Clinical Oncology*.[6] (A quality-adjusted year is a measure that allows researchers to factor in quality as well as quantity of life when calculating the value of a treatment.)

More than one-quarter of the cancer drugs under development are being tested broadly for their value against solid malignant tumors, the masses that grow in the breasts, prostate, lungs, and other organs. Others take aim at specific cancers—98 for cancers of the lung, 91 for breast cancer, 80 for prostate cancer, 63 for skin cancer, 55 for colorectal cancer, 49 for ovarian cancer, and 41 for pancreatic cancer.[7]

If the recent past is any example, very few of these are likely to represent major therapeutic breakthroughs. However, that won't stop the pharmaceutical industry from marketing them enthusiastically to physicians, including oncologists, and their patients. The drug companies go to great lengths to create awareness of new drugs and make their products seem appealing.

One avenue is television and magazine advertisements. That's known as "direct-to-consumer advertising," and it has been rapidly growing since the early 1990s. From 1996 to 2005, drug company spending on consumer advertising jumped by 330 percent, from $985 million to $4.24 billion.[8]

Asked in several surveys about the impact of such advertising, physicians generally indicated that the ads did a better job informing their patients about potential benefits than about possible risks. Of the surveyed physicians, 65 percent felt that the ads confused their patients about the tradeoffs between a drug's risks and its benefits, and 75 percent felt that patients believed a drug was more effective than it actually was.[9]

The pharmaceutical companies also woo doctors with "gifts." The retail value of the free samples they dispense approached $18.5 billion in 2005. Another $7.2 billion was spent that year on various forms of marketing and promotion, much of it on a practice called detailing, in which pharmaceutical representatives make sales calls to physician offices.[10] Ostensibly intended to educate providers, detailing can easily slide into a more overt effort to influence medical practice.

The industry also provides an array of other perks, including continuing education classes, consultant fees, and breakfasts and lunches for medical staff, to make health care professionals aware of what's on the market or in the pipeline.

"The pharmaceutical industry is interested in profit. They talk about research, but much of it is trying to persuade doctors to use their products," explains Mt. Sinai School of Medicine's Dr. James Holland.

An article in the *Journal of the American Medical Association* called the resulting "financial conflicts of interests . . . challenging and extensive" and was blunt about their possible impact on treatment decisions. "Research in the psychology and social science of gift receipt and giving indicates that current controls will not satisfactorily protect the interests of patients," said the authors. Instead, they advocated more-stringent regulations to modify a host of standard promotional practices—among them drug samples, continuing medical education, and reimbursement for travel expenses.[11]

The Business of Cancer Care

Regardless of any new rules designed to limit the relations between health care providers and the pharmaceutical industry, cancer drugs will remain big business.

KPMG, an international audit, tax, and advisory services firm, predicts that oncology drugs will provide the biggest source of growth for the entire industry, according to a 2011 report. Those revenues are expected to rise by an estimated 5 to 8 percent from 2010 to 2015, reaching $75 billion to $80 billion annually. The contribution of other major therapeutic classes to overall industry revenues pales by comparison. For example, diabetes drugs will likely grow by about 4 to 7 percent, with annual revenues in 2015 estimated to be $43 billion to $48 billion. Drugs to treat asthma and chronic obstructive pulmonary disorders are expected to generate $41 billion to $46 billion, based on a growth rate of 2 to 5 percent.[12]

Recognizing how lucrative the market can be, most major drug companies have invested substantially in cancer. Four targeted cancer drugs generated $8.4 billion in worldwide sales in 2005.[13] Three of these are produced by Swiss pharmaceutical giant Roche: rituximab (Rituxan), used to treat non-Hodgkin's lymphoma and rheumatoid arthritis; trastuzumab (Herceptin), which targets HER-2 positive breast cancer and metastatic stomach cancer; and bevacizumab (Avastin), used against many kinds of advanced cancers. The fourth engine of profits among these top sellers is imatinib mesylate (Gleevec), produced by Novartis and used to treat chronic myeloid leukemia.

Celgene, another global pharmaceutical giant, had earnings of almost $936 million in 2010, substantially driven by several oncology products. These include lenalidomide (Revlimid) and thalidomide (Thalomid), both used against multiple myeloma; azacitidine (Vidaza), for myelodysplastic syndromes, a pre-leukemic condition; and paclitaxel (Abraxane), to treat breast, lung, and ovarian cancers.[14]

In its annual report, Celgene was candid about the importance of its cancer drugs, noting that "a significant decline in demand for or use of these products or our other commercially available products could materially and adversely affect our operating results."

Celgene's frank observations reflect the reality that drug research and development is an expensive and risky undertaking, and it can be many years before a promising find pays off in a marketable therapy. A drug moves slowly from the laboratory to animal testing to three phases of human trials before a company is ready to navigate the complex process of FDA approval. If it is successful, development costs will likely have run anywhere from $1 billion to as much as $1.8 billion.

Often, the company doesn't reach that point. Only about 5 to 10 percent of potential cancer drugs survive the arduous journey from bench to bedside. About half of new cancer drugs fail the critical phase III clinical trials, when they are tested on the largest number of patients.[15] That means that at many points in the process, hope can turn to disappointment, and the drug companies will be back at the starting line.

Nonetheless, the fact that research is onerous does not excuse the industry for gouging consumers when it finds a winner. Companies are entitled to make a fair profit, but they also have an obligation to be good corporate citizens. "There is a special duty when you are selling medicine, as opposed to pantyhose or hubcaps," said Arthur Caplan, director of the Center for Bioethics at the University of Pennsylvania, in an interview with an online journal of the Wharton School of Business.[16]

One way that drug companies sustain their profits is through the US patent system. Theoretically, patent protections provide the exclusive right to market a product for a period of 20 years. In practice, because drugs are so slow to move from the lab to the patient, and because companies apply for a patent early in the development process, the effective patent period is about 11 years.[17] That is still a long and lucrative time to hold a monopoly—and is why the pharmaceutical industry is the most profitable industry in America. Twelve US pharmaceutical companies are on the Fortune 500 list of America's largest corporations. Annual revenue at Johnson and Johnson, which ranks 33rd, is almost $62 billion. Pfizer, Abbott Laboratories, and Merck are in the top 100 as well.[18]

The theory of patent protection is that exclusivity allows a company to recoup at least part of its investment on brand-name drugs before less expensive generic forms enter the marketplace. The competitive advantage that patents provide is also supposed to give companies an incentive to devote a large amount of funding to ambitious research.

The problem is that without competition, pharmaceutical companies can attach whatever price they want to anticancer agents. They do just that.

At $100,000 a year, Avastin may be the poster child for costly cancer drugs, and Genentech, now owned by Roche, made no apologies. Susan Desmond-Hellman, the president of product development at the time, said that Avastin's price is based on "the value of new innovation and the value of new therapies."[19] In essence, she argued that Genentech chose its price based on what the market would bear.

"She is only playing by the rules in a free-market society," observes John Marshall, MD, chief of the division of Hematology and Oncology at Georgetown University Hospital.

Genentech is far from alone. GlaxoSmithKline's ofatumumab

(Arzerra), used to treat chronic lymphocytic leukemia, costs $16,000 for a one-month course of treatment. One week of treatment with Genzyme's clofarabine (Clolar) for pediatric leukemia could run $34,000.[20]

Whatever we consider a reasonable cost for new cancer drugs, it would be hard to argue that that kind of pricing is fair, and it is certainly unsustainable.

RISING COSTS, SUSPECT SHORTAGES

Many other factors play a role in boosting the price of cancer drugs. When Congress created Medicare Part D, the prescription drug benefit, it specifically barred the Centers for Medicare and Medicaid (CMS) from negotiating reduced prices. That was an unusual step— one promoted by lobbyists—because the pharmaceutical industry routinely *does* negotiate with other segments of the federal government, as well as with private health plans. The Department of Veterans Affairs gets discounts, for example, paying an average of 48 percent less than Medicare for the 10 most frequently prescribed drugs.[21]

The inability to negotiate better drug prices for the huge pool of Medicare beneficiaries puts more stress on an already stressed system. Medicare covered 42.5 million people in 2005 and will cover some 70 million by 2030—and most of them will be over age 65, the population that's most vulnerable to cancer.[22]

A 2008 study published in the *Journal of the National Cancer Institute* gave a hint of what this will mean as the population grows old.[23] Researchers looked at a decade of Medicare records covering more than 306,000 people 65 and older, who had been diagnosed with breast, lung, colorectal, or prostate cancer. Those four cancers represent about 60 percent of the cancers that occur in older people.

The jump in the cost of their drugs, radiation, and surgical care was huge. In 1991, Medicare paid an average of about $7,100 for the initial treatment of lung cancer (defined as care provided in the first year after diagnosis); the comparable cost of treatment rose to almost $40,000 by the end of 2002. Yet survival rates have not improved.

Likewise, Medicare paid out just over $5,300 to treat one case of colorectal cancer in 1991 and more than $41,000 per patient a little more than a decade later. Early treatment for each breast cancer patient cost about $4,200 in 1991 and almost $21,000 in 2002. Only prostate cancer saw a tiny drop, falling by about $200, to $18,300, in the same period.

As a society, we simply cannot afford costs that soar by 500 percent or more in 10 years.

———

Recently, shortages of chemotherapy drugs have been another contributor to high costs, and a particularly unseemly one. Most of the shortages have occurred among generic drugs that have been on the market for years. "The main cause of drug shortages is economic," wrote Mandy L. Gatesman, of the Virginia Commonwealth University Health System, and Thomas J. Smith, MD, of Johns Hopkins University, in the *New England Journal of Medicine*.[24] If a manufacturer is not making substantial profits, or has an option of substituting a brand-name product that generates more revenues, they contend, the company will simply halt production of the generic alternative.

Their article includes a telling table that compares the average wholesale price of drugs in short supply with their more costly alternatives. For example, the generic drug paclitaxel, used to treat breast, lung, and ovarian cancer, is priced at $312 per dose—when it is available. A different formulation, no more effective and available only as a brand-name version called Abraxane, costs $5,800 per dose. Likewise, leucovorin, a generic drug to treat pediatric cancers and colon cancer, costs $32 per dose, while Fusilev, a close cousin that is no more effective, costs almost $1,300 per dose. Eight months after the FDA approved Fusilev, leucovorin was in short supply.

"There is a pattern here," Otis Brawley, MD, chief medical officer of the American Cancer Society, told *U.S. News and World Report*. "The drugs for which there is a shortage are the generic drugs, where the ability to make money is not as great."[25]

HOW PHYSICIANS PUSH UP COST

While part of the blame for soaring costs rests with the drug industry, oncologists must shoulder some responsibility as well. Patients or their insurers typically purchase chemotherapy drugs in the offices of their oncologists, and according to Gatesman and Smith's *New England Journal of Medicine* article, the sale of those drugs can account for more than half of the medical office's revenue.[26]

Much of that revenue is generated through Medicare reimbursement. For a long time, the CMS reimbursed oncologists for outpatient chemotherapy drugs on the basis of their wholesale prices (reimbursement rates were set at 95 percent of the wholesale price until 2004, when they were lowered to 85 percent of wholesale). Physicians could actually purchase the drugs far below wholesale, so Medicare provided them with a steady and sizable revenue stream.[27]

In 2005, Medicare shifted to a reimbursement structure based on the sales price oncologists were actually charged by the drug companies, and their margin of profit for chemotherapy fell sharply. Under the new system, CMS paid physicians only a 6 percent markup over the average sales price. The impact varied widely, as illustrated by reimbursement rates for three popular drugs used to treat a number of different cancers. Paclitaxel reimbursement plummeted from almost $2,270 to $225 for the standard monthly dose, while carboplatin fell by nearly half, from $1,845 to $930. By contrast, the change in reimbursement for docetaxel was minimal, falling from $2,732 to $2,506.

Predictably, the use of both paclitaxel and carboplatin declined afterward. "Physicians were prescribing these drugs to a smaller share of chemotherapy-treated patients than before because there was far less financial inducement to use them," Mireille Jacobson, a senior health economist at RAND, and her colleagues wrote in *Health Affairs*.[28] At the same time, prescriptions for the much more costly docetaxel increased modestly.

The logic is obvious. Oncologists stand to make a lot more money when they are getting an extra 6 percent for drugs that cost thousands of dollars, not a few hundred dollars or less.

"Where is the money in practicing oncology if you're in private practice? It's in administering chemotherapy," says Lora Weiselberg, MD, an oncologist and director of the Breast Cancer Service of the Don Monti Division of Medical Oncology at North Shore University Hospital in Manhasset, New York. "There is an incentive to prescribe more expensive drugs if you are going to profit from them. There is an inclination to use drugs that are going to benefit you more financially."

Many oncologists object to the idea that they are making decisions on the basis of their financial gain and insist that there is another side to the story. "I am sure there are doctors who prescribe expensive meds because they make more money than if they don't," acknowledges the American Society of Clinical Oncology's Dr. Nicholas Vogelzang. "I also know equally smart, even smarter doctors who go out of their way to give the most cost-effective medicines."

Certainly, it is not just revenue that drives oncologists' prescribing behavior. They are also influenced by the norms of medical training. Physicians have a passionate desire to find treatments that will work; it's fundamental to how we see ourselves as professionals. We know that medicine is very individual, and there is variation in the way in which patients respond to specific treatments. Even if research shows that a costly drug typically offers only a marginal benefit, we know that a small subset of the population is likely to respond better than the statistics suggest.

Perhaps, an oncologist thinks, my patient will be one of the lucky ones. Perhaps experimenting with two or more therapies might help, even if the combination has not been tested. When there are no other alternatives, oncologists on the front lines are understandably willing to give almost anything a try.

All this can be traced back to the core principle of medicine, as laid out in the Hippocratic Oath: the physician's pledge to apply medical knowledge to the treatment of the sick. At least that is how Ezekiel Emanuel, MD, PhD, chair of the department of medical ethics and health policy at the University of Pennsylvania, frames the issue. The problem, he points out, is that too often that translates into "an imperative to do everything for the patient regardless of cost or effect on others."[29]

He believes physicians should start thinking more about the consequences of that behavior. "We're the people who write the prescriptions. The pharmaceutical industry does not write the prescriptions," he says. "So why are we writing the prescriptions? Should we control ourselves better? We haven't done a tremendous job of thinking this through."

Unless doctors themselves take more responsibility for prescribing patterns that push up costs without doing much good, Dr. Emanuel says, regulators will likely take the initiative out of their hands.

I have tremendous respect for my medical colleagues, and I would like to see them participating in crafting solutions rather than adding to the problem. That means more than just offering another new drug of minimal value to a patient under their care. It means also thinking about the impact on society and of the greater good.

OTHER COST DRIVERS

Another factor driving the price of treatment is the American health insurance system, which generally covers most approved drugs, regardless of their price.

"We have health insurance, and health insurance evolved to be something that pays for drugs," says Georgetown University's Dr. Marshall. "As long as somebody else is paying, it doesn't matter how much they are." The result is an inelastic demand for drug treatment—consumption is not significantly altered by higher costs.

Health economist Scott Ramsey believes that a "cancer taboo," driven in part by well-organized advocacy groups and the threat of patient lawsuits, makes health insurers reluctant to deny coverage for any cancer treatment, regardless of its value. As a result, Ramsey wrote in the *Journal of Clinical Oncology,* "public and private health insurers make their adjustments in other places where the wheels aren't so squeaky."[30]

Insurance makes decisions related to health different from the decisions to purchase other consumer products, Dr. Marshall claims. He offers his suit-buying habits as an analogy.

Favoring Nordstrom, he often goes there to admire the fine cut of suits that run $1,800 or more. When it comes to making a purchase, though, he'll go to one of the discount stores where the suits are made of fabrics that are a bit less fine but have a nice fit all the same, and cost many hundreds of dollars less. "The point is that when I am shopping with my own money, I make a different decision, a different value judgment, than if I am shopping with someone else's money," he said in an interview with *Medscape* editor Bret Stetka, MD.[31]

Economists call this "moral hazard," the risk that individuals will behave differently because they are not paying for the costs of their behavior.

If the newest and most costly medicines were always the best ones, the issue here would be very different. We might be willing to allow only wealthy people to purchase pricey suits, but most of us would not be comfortable with a system that allows only the rich to have exclusive access to top-of-the-line health care. We would likely agree that insurers should keep paying so that everyone can have access to the best treatment.

With cancer care, the equivalent of a discount suit may be as good as the $1,800 version. If so, is it reasonable to expect public and private insurers to pay for the higher-priced cancer drug? The problem is that we have separated cost considerations from the evaluation of quality.

"In our health care system, we want freedom and access without the bill at the end of the day," says Dr. Marshall. "As professional consumers in America, we want more. More is better, we think. We have access to it; someone else is paying. It just creates a real cycle that drives up drug costs."

Certain therapeutic trends also influence costs. One culprit is the off-label use of cancer drugs.[32] After a drug has been approved by the FDA, physicians are allowed to prescribe it for any medical purpose they choose, regardless of what the label says. The logic has always been that the FDA does not regulate the practice of medicine, leaving physicians free to use a drug as they see fit, as long as it has demonstrated its safety and effectiveness for at least one condition.

The result is that we have oncologists treating breast cancer with a drug approved for colorectal cancer, or mixing and matching therapies that have not been tested together. Understandably desperate to find alternatives for gravely ill patients, oncologists generally resort to these untested strategies only when approved alternatives have failed them. It's an approach rooted in compassion, but it is expensive, it often carries serious side effects, and there may be little or no rigorous clinical data collected along the way. We aren't building knowledge from their informal experiments. Federal legislation requires Medicare to reimburse the cost of many drugs used off-label, but all too often we have no way of assessing whether they actually work.

Another pressure on costs comes from the oncology norm of using two or more anticancer drugs in combination, based on the theory that they may be more potent together. That's always a more expensive approach, but it is not always better medicine.

To assess the benefits, drugs that are going to be used in combination have traditionally first been studied and approved separately. Before licensing a single therapy that combines two approved drugs in a fixed dose, the FDA generally requires new studies to demonstrate that the combination is superior to either drug alone, as well as to the treatments that are currently considered the standard of care.

In a new trend, the industry is beginning to co-develop drug combinations, testing two novel therapies together to see how well they work. In contrast to the usual approach, neither drug has been approved, and neither may ever be used alone.

Co-developed drugs are part of the promising realm of targeted therapy research that takes aim against specific molecular characteristics of a tumor. Designed to strike at several cellular targets simultaneously, combination products are intended to do a better job of eluding the capacity of cancer cells to develop resistance.

For various technical reasons, it is often impossible to assess the individual therapeutic components of a co-developed product independently, creating challenges to the FDA's approval process. Whatever the promise of co-development, the regulatory agency is concerned enough about its risks to urge that it be used only for serious and life-threatening diseases that lack good treatment alternatives.

Nonetheless, the pharmaceutical companies see a potential new source of revenue here. The global management consulting firm Oliver Wyman candidly positioned novel drug combinations as an innovative way to compete "in the oncology marketplace" and said they could "justify premium pricing": "From the manufacturer's point of view, the correct price point could be as much as double the price of a single agent in order to get a return on investment equivalent to or beyond the value of developing two novel agents individually."

After consulting with insurance experts, Oliver Wyman was able to reassure the pharmaceutical industry that the premium price would likely be tolerable, at least for the moment. In its report, the firm declared, "For the time being, in the United States, if manufacturers demand significantly higher prices for dual-novel combos, health plans are likely to reimburse them."[33]

So it will go on unless we bring prevention to the forefront. Until then, we will all bear the burden of an unending spiral of rising costs.

CHAPTER 6

PAYING MORE, SETTLING FOR LESS

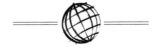

TIME AFTER TIME, WE HAVE GREETED NEW cancer treatments enthusiastically, only to discover that they offer the most marginal of benefits in exchange for serious side effects and a very high price tag. We keep spending more and more to provide cancer care, but we have not markedly improved quality. We seem far too willing to settle for less.

Colorectal cancer offers a startling example of some of the things that are wrong with our current emphasis on costly therapies for late-stage cancer that buy very little extra time. It is the third most common cancer in the United States, and the American Cancer Society estimates that in 2012 more than 100,000 people will be diagnosed with the disease and more than 50,000 people will die of it. Only lung cancer kills more people.[1]

In the 1990s, two chemotherapy drugs, fluorouracil and leu-covorin, were the standard combination treatment for colorectal cancer. Like other toxic drugs, they destroy normal cells that divide rapidly—including hair follicles, the lining of the gastrointestinal tract, and bone marrow—along with cancer cells. The price tag for 6 months of therapy: less than $100.[2] With these drugs, patients whose cancer has spread beyond the original site will live an average of 12 months longer than those who don't take them. So the drugs are affordable, but their value is limited.

Pharmaceutical researchers started looking for alternatives, and over the past decade they brought six significant new drugs to market, each with a tongue-twisting name and a different mode of action. Capecitabine (Xeloda), an oral form of fluorouracil, is an antimetabolite, designed to stop or slow the growth of cancer cells. Irinotecan (Camptosar), part of a class of antineoplastic medications called topoisomerase I inhibitors, also stops cancer cells from growing. Oxaliplatin (Eloxatin) is a platinum-containing antineoplastic agent that kills cancer cells.

The targeted therapies to treat colorectal cancer include three monoclonal antibodies: cetuximab (Erbitux), bevacizumab (Avastin), and panitumumab (Vectibix). These drugs, too, have different modes of action, either preventing growth-signaling activities, blocking growth receptors, or interfering with the steps necessary to initiate new blood vessels.

In various combinations, these drugs have the ability to lengthen life. For example, using the standard fluorouracil and leucovorin, plus two of the newer chemotherapy drugs, irinotecan and oxaliplatin, gave patients nine extra months to live, extending overall survival by up to 21 months.[3] Add some of the monoclonal antibodies, and patients often did slightly better.[4]

That good news comes with a huge price tag. Adding a dose of irinotecan every three weeks for six months to fluorouracil and leucovorin tacks $30,000 onto the bill (in 2004 dollars). Administering Avastin every other week costs $24,000 for a course of treatment. Erbitux is even pricier, with six months of weekly treatments topping $50,000.

Tally all the treatments typically given to a patient with metastatic colon cancer, and we are talking about a cost of $150,000 to $200,000, all for an additional year of survival. And that's the price tag for one patient with one cancer.[5]

———

The same scenario plays out across the cancer spectrum. Researchers keep looking for new treatment regimens, because not all cancers respond the same way to the same anticancer drugs, and most eventually develop resistance to even the most potent drugs.

Obviously, we need a better arsenal against cancer. When prevention has failed, lives can be extended with more effective cancer treatments. "If you have metastatic melanoma and it's in your liver and lungs and you're 30 years old, you tell me what 10 months is worth," says the American Society of Clinical Oncology's Dr. Nicholas Vogelzang.

Besides, statistics are in the end just guidelines and averages. When researchers say that a drug has an average survival benefit of six months, it usually means that one person may live just four months longer but another may gain eight or more extra months of life. The individual circumstances of every case obviously influence the outcome.

All this helps to explain why oncologists keep offering new therapies. Unfortunately, their desperate efforts often have a tragic result: Their patients endure their final weeks and months of life in misery—there is no other word to describe it.

We are spending huge sums of money to sustain that misery. Thirty percent of Medicare expenses cover the costs of the 5 percent of beneficiaries who die each year.[6] At the same time, we are dedicating the tiniest sums to palliative care, which acknowledges the reality of death and tries to make it as peaceful as possible by providing psychosocial support and managing symptoms, rather than toxic treatment.

In their final days, when cancer simply cannot be stopped, many people would prefer the palliative care option. Yet many oncologists, unwilling to admit that some of their patients are dying, never even raise the topic. An *Archives of Internal Medicine* study found that doctors had discussed hospice with only half of their metastatic lung cancer patients two months before their deaths.[7] Many patients are referred to hospice care only in the last few days of their lives, undermining some of its tremendous power to offer comfort.

These failures are a disservice to both patients and society. The costs of care for people who have end-of-life discussions can be considerably lower than for those who do not—and critically, their quality of life can be higher.[8] One study found that patients receiving palliative care were less depressed and lived an average of three months longer than those who received standard care.[9]

Despite this, the cancer culture continues to claim that new drugs with the most marginal of benefits are cause for celebration. Measures of "meaningful improvement" that should be unacceptable to us all are routinely assigned to patient outcomes.

A study published in the *Lancet* looked at what happens when the monoclonal antibody cetuximab is added to a standard two-drug regimen. Median survival rose from 10.1 months to 11.3 months, and the authors declared the combination "a new standard first-line treatment option."[10]

Technically, that was true. But the 18 weeks of treatment necessary to gain those extra 1.2 months of life cost an average of $80,000. At that rate, the cost to give a person one more year of life would be $800,000, according to an estimate published in the *Journal of the National Cancer Institute*.[11]

Taking that calculation one step further, the authors pointed out that if the same $800,000 could be spent to add a year to the lives of each of the 555,000 Americans who die of cancer every year, the bill would be $440 billion—nearly 100 times more than the National Cancer Institute's entire annual budget. And even then, they emphasized, "no one would be cured."

Such exorbitant price tags for such modest benefits are the rule rather than the exception. More than 90 percent of anticancer agents approved by the FDA between 2004 and 2009 cost more than $20,000 for 12 weeks of treatment.[12]

When the monoclonal antibody ipilimumab (Yervoy) reached the marketplace in 2011, it was hailed as a game changer for people with metastatic melanoma. Paired with a second drug, it extended life by just over 2 months (11.2 months versus 9.1 months).[13] At a price, of course. Bristol-Myers Squibb charged $120,000 for four infusions over 3 months.[14] That longer survival time may be torturous. Side effects of Yervoy can include a variety of inflammatory responses affecting the intestines, eyes, hormone-producing glands, and nerves. Some patients developed a perforated intestine or became paralyzed.[15]

Then there is the story of erlotinib (Tarceva), a monoclonal antibody that may have set a new low for improving life expectancy. Combining erlotinib and standard therapy to treat advanced pancreatic cancer extends survival by 6.2 months, compared with 5.9 months for standard treatment alone. That's a difference of approximately 10 days.

Yet, the authors of the article discussing erlotinib in the *Journal of Clinical Oncology* article treated this as a genuine enhancement, writing, "We found that overall survival in patients with advanced pancreatic cancer was significantly improved."[16]

THE PROGRESSION-FREE SURVIVAL THRESHOLD

Many drug therapies are not even studied on the basis of their impact on overall survival, but rather on their impact on progression-free survival or the maintenance of stable disease. There's a big difference.

The National Cancer Institute defines progression-free disease as "the length of time during and after treatment in which a patient is living with a disease that does not get worse." Its definition of stable disease is similar: "cancer that is neither decreasing or increasing in extent or severity."

"Progression-free survival is how long a treatment works before the tumor starts to grow again," explains North Shore University

Hospital's Dr. Lora Weiselberg. "Survival is how long you live."

The ultimate goal, of course, is longer survival. Yet we have come to accept progression-free survival as if it were something to applaud. The shift in our thinking can be traced back to one of the few therapies that did turn one type of cancer into a chronic and manageable disease.[17]

That was Gleevec, the monoclonal antibody that transformed the lives of people diagnosed with chronic myeloid leukemia (CML). One study, published in the *Journal of the National Cancer Institute,* found that eight years after beginning treatment, patients with CML had a death rate that matched that of the general population. Researchers called Gleevec the "first drug to produce complete and lasting responses in CML patients" and said that it "offers the first evidence that a disseminated cancer not amenable to surgery can be controlled to the point of giving patients a normal life expectancy."[18]

The powerful long-term results of Gleevec reinforced the concept of treating cancer as a chronic disease, much like diabetes or hypertension. Without diminishing that success story, the special features of CML, which involves only a single genetic mutation, have so far made it unique. Solid tumors, such as cancers of the lung, brain, breast, and colon, are several orders of magnitude more complicated than CML.

Most of the drugs we have to fight solid tumors influence a specific part of a cellular cycle and have only a transient effect. They don't stop the progress of a tumor indefinitely. A slow-growing tumor is still growing and is perhaps beginning to spread undetected elsewhere in the body.

Unless we find radically different approaches, we can expect the trend of generating newer, more expensive cancer-fighting therapies, which aren't much better than the previous ones, to continue.

We can talk about progression-free survival, but the treatments we offer will not be able to help someone live much longer. If we don't shift our focus to prevention, and better methods of early detection, we'll still be faced with wily cancer cells that eventually outwit our most costly, cutting-edge treatments, whether they do so slowly or quickly. We'll still be trapped in a cycle of new drug development, followed by disappointment, ad infinitum. We'll keep on settling for less.

Some argue that accepting the status quo is exactly what we have to do, and that no matter how we define survival, or how much treatment it takes to maintain it, we should be content with controlling disease for as long as possible. From that vantage point, the more cancer treatments we have, the better off we are.

"There are many solid tumors that have a very poor prognosis," says Jerry Zeldis, MD, PhD, who is the CEO of Celgene Global Health, a pharmaceutical company. "Certain cancers will kill you right away, and others will make you suffer for a very long time. From my perspective, if there are agents that can prolong peoples' lives without disabling them, that's a wonderful thing."

Not everyone agrees. Mt. Sinai School of Medicine's legendary cancer researcher Dr. James Holland doesn't particularly care for the model of managing cancer as a chronic disease. "Good oncologists are interested in cancer prevention," he emphasizes.

Many cancer advocacy groups agree. In 2010, the National Breast Cancer Coalition set a deadline for ending breast cancer once and for all, announcing it with these stirring words:

Today we set a goal. Today we set a deadline. January 1, 2020. The end of breast cancer. Hope is a wish. The deadline is a commitment. Hope says whenever. The deadline says within ten years. What if we fail? We already have. What about pink? It's time to show our true colors. Ten years is too short? We ended polio in seven.

A deadline changes everything. No experiment, no charity, no lab, no doubt, no promise, no critic, no iota of research can occur outside of its context. Today the conversation changes. 2020. The end of breast cancer.[19]

Fran Visco, president of the National Breast Cancer Coalition, says, "I don't want to maintain the status quo. I don't want to just voice dissatisfaction with the status quo. I want to change it."

THE AVASTIN STORY

The American Society of Clinical Oncology hailed the monoclonal antibody Avastin, which inhibits the growth of blood cells in tumors, as a promising treatment for recurrent ovarian cancer. Its 2011 annual report described two clinical trials in which Avastin, combined with standard chemotherapy, "helped women with recurrent ovarian cancer live significantly longer without their disease worsening than those treated with the same chemotherapy alone."[20]

The word "significantly" had a statistical meaning that was far from the urgently needed breakthrough it implied. In one clinical trial described in the report, women lived a median of four months longer before their cancer progressed.

These results were essentially confirmed in studies published in the *New England Journal of Medicine.* One reported that adding Avastin to the treatment of women with ovarian cancer while they were also receiving chemotherapy, or up to 10 months afterward, extended progression-free survival by a median of about 4 months.[21] The other study measured the effect of a different regimen of chemotherapy plus Avastin and found a 2-month improvement in progression-free survival.[22]

Although all this was framed as good news, the marginal benefits of Avastin were exorbitantly priced, at up to $100,000 per year.[23] In addition, the side effects could be horrendous, including gastrointestinal perforation, sometimes fatal bleeding, slow or incomplete wound healing, and stroke or heart attack. In fact, these side effects led the FDA to revoke its approval of Avastin to treat metastatic breast cancer in late 2011.[24]

Three years earlier, Roche had received accelerated approval for that indication under the FDA's fast-track system, reserved for promising drugs to treat life-threatening conditions that lack alternative therapies. That approval was based on a finding that Avastin combined with the chemotherapy drug paclitaxel extended progression-free survival by an average of 11.8 months, compared with 5.9 months for women treated with paclitaxel alone.[25]

The logic for the accelerated approval was understandable. There was a desperate need for new treatment options, plus tremendous excitement about the drug. When drugs are approved on an accelerated basis, research is supposed to continue, and the next round of studies showed a much more modest impact. The survival advantage of Avastin fell to somewhere between less than 1 month and less than 3, depending on the study. Based on the new evidence, the FDA concluded that Avastin's risks did not justify its limited benefits for metastatic breast cancer.

Although the FDA's approval about-face was controversial, especially among patients desperate for new treatments, many think it was the right thing to do. Fran Visco is among them. "The manufacturer of Avastin behaved badly when it pushed for its approval for the treatment of breast cancer, especially when the research indicated that Avastin wasn't working for breast cancer and that there was significant harm that the drug could do," she says.

Avastin is simply not a lifesaving drug, according to Clifford Hudis, MD, the chief of the Breast Cancer Medicine Service at Memorial Sloan-Kettering Cancer Center. "Progression-free survival is not survival. Avastin has not increased survival for any of these patients," he says.

Yet, this drug remains on the market, not only for ovarian cancer but for colon and lung cancer as well. (While doctors can prescribe approved drugs for any purpose, the FDA approves drugs for specific purposes, which can influence reimbursement decisions as well as the extent of a drug's clinical use.) More recent research suggests that the drug may be a useful treatment prior to breast cancer surgery, albeit with serious side effects, so the debate is far from settled.[26]

Still, the Avastin story is a cautionary tale. Too many stakeholders pushed too hard to bring a drug of questionable benefit, certain toxicity, and tremendous cost to market. As a January 2012 *New England Journal of Medicine* editorial reminds us, " . . . in the context of unsustainable expenditures for cancer care in the United States, any survival benefit of bevacizumab, or other molecularly targeted drugs must ultimately be balanced against their considerable costs."[27]

Too Little, Too Late

Toxic, expensive therapies with borderline advantages, or none at all, seem to be all we are offering patients with advanced cancer.

Nevertheless, we can't seem to break the habit of putting new drugs on the shelves, and oncologists just keep on prescribing them.

"The whole gestalt of our approach to cancer control is too dominated by the pharmaceutical companies," insists Lee Hartwell, PhD, who served as president of the Fred Hutchinson Cancer Research Center in Seattle for more than a decade, until 2010. In 2001, he won the Nobel Prize for discovering the genes that control cell division. "We ought to admit that this approach is not the panacea for cancer and have a much more balanced approach to the whole problem, where prevention and earlier detection have a much greater chance of providing benefit," he says.[28]

True, there are legitimate arguments for approving and using therapies that extend life ever so slightly in the sickest of patients. One is that marginal drugs may suggest mechanisms of action that point the way toward better treatment. "These minor steps in advanced cancer give us a clue that a drug actually does something," explains Dr. Vogelzang.

Also, while experimental therapies tend to be tried first in patients whom standard drugs have failed, they may ultimately prove much more effective in people with earlier-stage disease. "That is the nature of cancer medicine," Dr. Vogelzang says.

In practice, it doesn't work that way. In a provocative commentary in the *Journal of the National Cancer Institute,* Tito Fojo and Christine Grady noted that the hope of new drugs becoming stepping stones to improved treatment options often goes unrealized.[29] They said that we have not actually had much success at shifting drugs from use in metastatic disease to use as first-line treatment. "We should stop developing and approving therapies with marginal benefits in the advanced setting with the hopes of transforming them into curative regiments up-front," they wrote.

To expect this to prove useful is to "place hope above data, experience and reality."

―――

The United Kingdom takes a very different approach. Its National Institute for Health and Clinical Excellence (NICE) recommends drugs that the National Health Service (NHS) should pay for. NHS, the publicly funded health care system in the United Kingdom, wants to know: Are the benefits a drug provides worth the cost, in light of the side effects? NHS has "a flat budget," says Georgetown University's Dr. John Marshall. If NHS decides a new medicine is good and important, it might say, "We need to bring this in, but we'll have to get rid of what we don't use or is less effective," he explains.

Quite a few cancer drugs routinely used in the United States have not been approved in the United Kingdom because they aren't sufficiently cost-effective. An article in the *Journal of Clinical Oncology* looked at 59 cancer drugs approved in the United States from 2004 to 2008. The Centers for Medicare and Medicaid Services and the Department of Veterans Affairs reimbursed physicians who prescribed any of them. Forty-six of these drugs were also approved for use in the United Kingdom—but NICE would reimburse for only 18 of them (decisions about reimbursement for some of the others were pending at the time the research was published).[30]

Clearly, public officials in the United Kingdom have a different method for evaluating cancer treatments. An example is NICE's January 2012 recommendation not to pay for cabazitaxel (Jevtana) as a component of prostate cancer treatment. The drug did extend life, the agency concluded, but its adverse effects, especially diarrhea and some of the hematological consequences, did not justify reimbursing for its use.

Sir Andrew Dillon, the chief executive officer of NICE, explained, "The independent Committee appraising this drug concluded that it would not provide enough health benefit to justify its cost, which means it would not be a cost effective use of limited NHS resources."[31]

NICE has also recommended against all three monoclonal antibodies available in the United States to treat advanced colorectal cancer, including Avastin. In reaching its decisions, NICE made very explicit cost calculations. Estimating that 6,500 people a year would be eligible for Avastin, and that Roche was asking the NHS to pay approximately £20,800 (about $33,000) per patient, the cost could be as high as £135 million (about $214 million).

Paying that much to give 6,500 patients an average of six weeks more of life was just not justified, in NICE's view. "There were simply too many uncertainties in the economic analysis to be able to recommend the drug for use in the NHS," the institute declared.[32]

Likewise, NICE has been less than enthusiastic about Yervoy, the much-ballyhooed drug for melanoma. NICE says the drug is too costly, its long-term benefits are not fully known, and it generates adverse reactions that can "significantly affect a patient's quality of life."[33]

Americans are much more reluctant to acknowledge these kinds of tradeoffs. We pretend that we can afford to pay for everything, no matter how minimal the benefit. "In England, they are sacrificing real, but small, survival advantages," says Dr. Marshall.

What is acceptable in the United Kingdom's public health care system would likely raise the specter of "death panels" here if Medicare tried to deny coverage for some approved products. We saw that kind of rhetoric when Congress proposed to reimburse physicians for having end-of-life discussions with their patients, and it would surely surface again in any conversation that drew a line between drugs that are valuable enough to pay for and those that are not.

"Value is not part of our official medical language," Dr. Marshall said in a *Medscape* interview. He pointed out that the FDA's approval process is based only on a drug's safety and effectiveness, not on its cost, and that the Center for Medicare and Medicaid Services is expected to pay for any drug the FDA approves. "We are the only country with 'modern' medicine that does not include a value element in this process." [34]

The University of Pennsylvania's Dr. Ezekiel Emanuel agrees, adding bluntly, "We should differentiate between drugs that make a small difference and drugs that make no difference at all. A lot of cancer drugs are not worth very much in terms of prolongation of life."

In the United States, the establishment of the Patient-Centered Outcomes Research Institute is one hopeful step toward basing health care decisions on rigorous evidence of what works. Created under the 2010 health care reform legislation, it is a science-based research approach designed to help patients and their health care providers make the best possible medical decisions.

Unfortunately, the legislation that created the Patient-Centered Outcomes Research Institute continues the tradition of ignoring the limits of our resources. It explicitly bars the institute from considering costs as it compares different ways to achieve good health outcomes. Once more, we are refusing to address the issues of value, cost-effectiveness, and sustainability in health care.

We do this because we are uncomfortable with explicitly denying access to some costly treatments, and yet we actually do just that—even though we are not very candid about it.

"We are rationing treatments now based on insurance coverage," says Dr. Marshall. Under the current health care system, patients who can't afford the co-payments required by their insurance are sometimes forced to change medications or to resort to even riskier practices, such as reducing their dosages or skipping a medicine altogether.

Doctors also make treatment recommendations that are driven by what insurance will cover and their patients' resources. "My patients think they are all getting the same 'best' standard of care, but I am prescribing different medicines to different patients based on their health care plans," Dr. Marshall acknowledges. "It is rationing, in a sense."

If most therapies worked well for most patients—whether or not they actually cured the disease—we could accept their value, even as we try to foster a hard societal discussion about how to afford them. That's not the situation we have now. Many of these therapies are at once breathtakingly expensive, brutal in their side effects, and lacking in long-term advantages. That should tell us we have headed off course.

CHAPTER 7

CANCER'S COLLATERAL DAMAGE

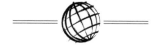

ANYONE WHO HEARS THE TERRIFYING WORDS "you have cancer" likely does not focus first on what treatment will cost. Catapulted into self-preservation mode by the news, most people embark instead on a search for the most powerful cancer-fighting tools they can find, and all too often that becomes a search that never ends. The "I'll try anything and worry about costs later" approach has become the default mode.

The problem is all the collateral damage that results.

PAYING THE PRICE

Toni and Doug's journey through cancer speaks volumes about that. Toni, a 50-year-old artist, and Doug, a 50-year-old golf professional, saw the darkest side of our current cancer care paradigm. The couple endured Toni's frequent hospitalizations, the debilitating side effects of one cancer drug after another, false hope, and a mounting pile of bills. Their ordeal ended with Toni's death four years after her diagnosis of lymphoma.

The story began in September 2007, at the end of a hard day working on a major project in their yard. Doug noticed a walnut-size lump on the inside of his wife's left thigh.

"It's just a bruise," Toni told him. "It'll go away."

Two weeks later, it was still there, and two other lumps had appeared in her groin area. They were the size of marbles, but painless. Toni saw a nurse practitioner, who agreed that the lump on her leg was probably just a bruise and recommended treating it with warm compresses. The nurse thought the groin lumps were more likely to be hernias and advised Toni to consult a surgeon.

In late November, after the lumps had been biopsied, her doctors delivered the devastating news that they were malignant. Toni was diagnosed with diffuse large B-cell lymphoma, a common form of non-Hodgkin's lymphoma.

Scans revealed that Toni had an especially aggressive cancer, with tumors scattered across her lower abdominal area and elsewhere. Still, her oncologists spoke optimistically about the package of treatment options available, and she was cooperative and prepared for the fight. After surgery to remove the tumors, Toni began a six-cycle regimen of chemotherapy, receiving an eight-hour infusion every few weeks. By the third round, she could barely move from her bed between infusions, but she persevered, and at the end of June, the couple received good news. "We got it," her doctors proclaimed. Everyone believed the cancer was gone.

Toni was told she would have to return for scans every three months for the first year, and then less frequently. Doug remembers the doctor saying, "After five years, you won't have to come back at all."

Weakened by the chemotherapy, Toni spent much of the summer and fall regaining her strength. Life for the couple was good again.

Until March 2009, that is, when a post-treatment scan showed that the cancer had recurred and had spread. Toni's oncologist suggested that she would be a good candidate for a bone marrow transplant, which had to be done at a cancer center about 100 miles from their home.

After learning more about the rigorous and difficult procedure—including claims that it had a 95 percent success rate—Toni agreed to begin treatment.

Additional potent chemotherapy had to come first. This time, Toni was admitted to the local hospital, where she received chemo around the clock for three days every three weeks. A post-chemo scan again showed no evidence of cancer, and the couple headed to the cancer center, ready for the bone marrow transplant. Their insurance company had already said yes to the $400,000 treatment. It was July 2009.

The first step was to harvest Toni's bone marrow stem cells, which took eight hours a day over five consecutive days. Another week of chemotherapy came next, and then the stem cells were infused back into her body during a four-hour procedure.

She remained hospitalized for the next three weeks, as the stem cells started to grow again. Once, her blood pressure plunged and her platelet levels dropped to dangerously low levels, bringing her perilously close to death.

Although she recovered, Toni's health had been compromised, and remained so after her release from the hospital. Shortly afterward, her temperature spiked to 105°F, a fungal infection was found in her lungs, and she was readmitted for further treatment. The fungus might have been there for a long time, held in check until her immune system was weakened by chemotherapy and could no longer fight the latent infection. Her antifungal medicine cost $5,600 a month.

Toni was finally able to return home in late October, although the demands of continuing treatment and follow-up meant the couple had to make weekly four-hour round-trip drives to the hospital.

In February 2010, Toni returned for a scan, expecting it to show that the bone marrow transplant had worked. The couple thought this would be their moment of triumph, a second chance for a longer life. Instead, they learned that Toni still had evidence of cancer. A year of suffering and sacrifice had been in vain.

Her doctors suggested another transplant. Nothing else will work, they said. Toni balked. "No," she said. "You didn't have to go through what I went through. You didn't almost die. You're not the ones who didn't have any quality of life for almost a year."

Then, she added quietly, "I don't know whether or not we can afford it."

The doctors' response: "You don't have to worry. Your insurance company paid for everything the first time. It will pay for everything again."

That wasn't quite true, of course. "Insurance didn't pay for us to live away from home for eight months," Doug recalls. "It didn't pay for a lot of the drugs Toni needed. It didn't pay for the fact that both of us were out of work for quite some time. The insurance company covers the medical cost, but it doesn't cover the costs of the disease."

Even so, they decided to try another transplant. Over the next few months, more health problems intervened. Toni's spleen swelled to five times its normal size, her white blood cell count plunged, and she developed pneumonia. Meanwhile, scans showed that her cancer kept surging.

Still, the doctors insisted she remained a candidate for the transplant. The procedure was scheduled, canceled, rescheduled, and canceled once more.

As many patients do when they have exhausted all other options, Toni entered a clinical trial, this one assessing a new combination drug treatment. Beginning in April 2011, the couple began making regular trips to the hospital for the protocol. With the tumors shrinking, the punishing treatment schedule seemed worth it. The second bone marrow transplant again seemed possible.

Then, new obstacles arose. When Toni complained of headaches, invasive tests revealed that lymphoma cells had invaded her cerebral spinal fluid. The cancer was in her brain.

Yet another drug treatment option was put on the table, but this time her oncologist was finally ready to advise against it. "You can do this if you want, but I don't recommend it," he said bluntly. "You will be in the hospital for six months. It'll be hell, and then you will die."

Toni's fight was over. The doctor said that she would probably survive until Thanksgiving but doubted that she would make it to Christmas. On September 29, 2011, Toni's courageous four-year battle came to an end. She was 54.

When illness first occurred, Toni and Doug had steady jobs, good insurance, and friends willing to help. Financially, they were luckier than many. After they had met their annual $4,500 deductible, their health insurance had paid out more than $1 million. Pharmaceutical companies provided some of Toni's medications for free through patient assistance programs. At the golf course where Doug works, colleagues and friends raised nearly $50,000 to cover some of their expenses.

Yet Doug knows he won't be retiring anytime soon. The couple incurred $50,000 in out-of-pocket medical costs and another $150,000 in living expenses, including bills for hotels, food, and gas. After long periods without a regular income, the couple couldn't meet their monthly obligations. They tapped savings accounts, used credit cards, sold stocks when the market was down, and took out an equity line of credit on their home. Decades of careful savings vanished.

Doug is not a bitter man, but he has mixed feelings about what they endured. "I was not going to tell Toni to give up," he says. "It was her choice. There were nights when she was in so much pain. I'd say, 'Honey, if you are ready to go, it's fine.'" But Toni did not want to die. She wrote a book about her struggle to inform and inspire other cancer patients, and she still hoped to beat the cancer, to see her daughter married, to hold her first grandchild.

Doug wonders now if they were given false hope. "Had we known the full extent of what was ahead, I don't think we would have gone through what we did," he says.

"At some point, the hope isn't realistic. Do I think we needed to go through the last year we went through? No, I don't. Toni was treated at a teaching hospital. Was what we went through done to teach somebody else? Or was it done for the revenue? I hope it wasn't. I hope it was done more to teach the people there. Was it for Toni's benefit? I'm not entirely sure it was."

It is hard for him not to feel cynical about the agenda of those in the cancer industry and the influence of money on decision making. "In my heart, I believe if we wanted to find a cure for cancer, we would have done so a long time ago," he says. "I don't believe the medical profession wants to find a cure. They would like to find effective treatments for cancer, but a cure? No. There would be too many people out of work."

Doug is particularly rankled by the silence from Toni's oncologist and other cancer care providers after her death. They did not reach out to him with words of comfort or respect. "I am sorry, but if you have been to someone more than 180 times over four years and you have contributed to the well-being of their office, I think a card is appropriate. I think it's appropriate to say, 'Your wife put up a hell of a fight. You did everything you could.'

"I truly believe," he adds, "that if our insurance hadn't paid the doctors as well as it did, they wouldn't have encouraged us to keep on with treatment."

———

Understandably, Doug may be a bit harsh in his judgment of Toni's physicians. Treating people with cancer is a delicate and tricky process, with oncologists trying to keep their patients alive by staying one step ahead of the disease. It is hard to know just how much extra gain can be achieved, at what price, and exactly when the struggle becomes futile.

Right now, most therapy buys patients with advanced cancer only a little more time. Oncologists are often trying their best to honor a patient's wishes when they keep suggesting new options. Although those haunting words about the willingness to "place hope above data, experience, and reality" come to mind, this is what medicine trains physicians to do, and it is a mission they believe in.

"It is emotionally draining," admits Dr. Nicholas Vogelzang, chair of the American Society of Clinical Oncology's Cancer Communications Committee. "But you have the privilege of really getting to know your patients. That's an honor reserved for rabbis, priests, and pastors. That is why being a physician is a sacred calling. I honestly think the reward is the work and the benefit you give the patient and the family."

He quotes a line from the Talmud, the authoritative guide to Jewish law and ethics: "Whoever destroys a soul, it is considered as if he destroyed an entire world. And whoever saves a life, it is considered as if he saved an entire world."

That, Dr. Vogelzang says, "is the underpinning of why we treat cancer and why we constantly strive to find better therapies."

COSTS WE CANNOT AFFORD

Still, the impact of high costs on patients, their families, and the entire society cannot be ignored. As Toni and Doug discovered, there are many unexpected expenses associated with cancer, including diagnostics and treatments that are not reimbursed; the premiums, deductibles, and co-payments required by many plans; the loss of wages; and the expenses of traveling long distances for state-of-the-art care. That's without even trying to set a price for quality-of-life losses, strain on caregivers, and the terrible toll the disease takes on a network of beloved friends and family.

In a national survey of adults in 1,000 households affected by cancer, the Kaiser Family Fund reported that 25 percent said they had used up all or most of their savings, and 11 percent said they were unable to pay for basic necessities, such as food, heat, or housing.[1] The survey also found that families are making life-and-death decisions based on pocketbook issues—8 percent of families surveyed said that a family member with cancer had delayed getting care, or decided not to get it at all, because of the cost.

Having insurance is obviously vital, but even that is no guarantee against financial hardship. Nearly one-quarter of those surveyed said their insurance had paid less than they anticipated for a bill, and 10 percent said they had reached the cap on their insurance coverage for cancer, meaning they would not continue to be reimbursed for cancer treatment.

A study in the *Journal of Oncology Practice* illustrates how costs can influence a patient's medical choices. Researchers examined the use of oncolytic therapy, an expensive and relatively new class of cancer drugs designed to destroy tumor cells and deliver antitumor genes to the body. Oncolytic therapy has the advantage of being administered orally, rather than through an intravenous drip.[2]

The study found that some people discontinued use of this medication after initially filling a prescription, presumably once they discovered what their out-of-pocket costs would be. The "abandonment rate" was about 10 percent, and patients who had to pay more than $500 of their own money were four times more likely to abandon it than those who incurred costs of $100 or less.

Other evidence of the burdensome costs of cancer comes from the federal Agency for Healthcare Research and Quality. Its research found that 13 percent of individuals under age 55 with cancer were likely to spend more than 20 percent of their total income on all health care services (including insurance-related expenses). The highest burden fell on those with private, individual coverage (43 percent of that group spent more than 20 percent of their total income on cancer coverage and care).[3]

Startling numbers also show that in the United States, adults on Medicare can pay as much as $6,000 out of their own pockets for therapies that the National Health Service in the United Kingdom will not pay for at all because they offer such marginal benefits.[4]

A cancer diagnosis increases the likelihood of personal bankruptcy. In research presented at the 2011 meeting of the American Society of Clinical Oncology, Dr. Scott Ramsey, the director of Cancer Outcomes Research at Seattle's Fred Hutchinson Cancer Research Center and a health economist, reported that people with cancer are about seven times more likely to file for bankruptcy than the general population. (That's an approximate comparison—according to Dr. Ramsey, 1.9 percent of patients are bankrupt within 5 years of a cancer diagnosis, compared with 0.28 percent of the general population over 10 years.)[5]

In still another wrenching example of what cancer can mean in economic terms, some patients are factoring in the financial impact on their families when they make treatment choices. As Paula Kim writes in the *Journal of Clinical Oncology*, "Some patients, with or without endorsement and acknowledgment from their loved ones, refuse to accept treatment that will saddle their families with unmanageable debt."[6] They may be particularly likely to forgo "optional" treatments, such as mental health services, end-of-life palliative care, and pain medication, to protect the family's solvency.

Are we really willing to let dying people go without pain relief in their final days of life because of the costs involved? Is that how we want to approach cancer in the 21st century?

Beyond the immediate impact on families, the consequences of cancer's high costs are ultimately felt by all of us.

Gregg, the long-term survivor of non-small cell lung cancer, recognized this as he reflected on his own treatment. For nine years, Gregg tried just about every standard and novel therapy on the market. The price, paid first by his private insurance company and then by Medicare, exceeded $2 million. "I hardly paid a cent out of pocket," he acknowledged.

While Gregg was grateful for that, he wondered how we as a society can afford it. That's a good question. To the extent that Medicare, Medicaid, and other public-sector programs cover costs, it means that we either raise taxes or allocate fewer dollars to other government investments. Less money is available for schools, transportation, infrastructure, environmental innovations, stimulating new business, supporting vulnerable populations, and so forth.

The use of private insurance to pay for cancer also carries social costs. Insurance companies don't make profits when they pay out more than they take in, so they compensate by raising premiums, lowering reimbursement to health care providers, cutting back on the benefits they offer—or doing all three. If premiums go up, employers may reduce the coverage they provide, or require more cost-sharing from employees. Employees, in turn, may drop coverage that's unaffordable.

Physicians are in an uncomfortable role here, being asked both to do their best for their patients and to take a stand on behalf of broader social concerns. Many do not consider pricing in their treatment decisions, and others are not inclined to shoulder responsibility for conserving the resources of public and private insurers.

In one survey, more than three-quarters of the physicians said that cost would not influence their inclination to prescribe Avastin, given that the FDA considered it effective enough to approve. Yet most felt the drug did not offer "good value for the money," based on its survival benefit and costs.[7]

Do their patients want that kind of drug? Many medical providers can't answer that question. Almost one-third of oncologists indicated in a survey that they felt uncomfortable discussing the costs of chemotherapy with their patients.[8]

"Physicians find themselves in an unusual and awkward position," says Memorial Sloan-Kettering Cancer Center's Dr. Clifford Hudis. "On the one hand, we are individual advocates for patients. On the other hand, we're being asked to be the judge and gatekeeper with regard to societal resources, like shared insurance money."

Another locus of responsibility rests with the pharmaceutical companies, and here, too, there is little consensus on how they should behave, what they should charge, and who should try to influence their behavior.

"I am perfectly happy with the high prices of drugs if you deliver high value to patients. Most drugs are a terrific bargain," claims Roy Vagelos, MD, the retired CEO and chairman of Merck. He acknowledges, however, that drugs need to offer meaningful benefits to justify their price. When the price of cancer drugs is "unrelated to the value they deliver to the patient," he says, "that is bad for the industry and terrible for society."

As we shift to a prevention model, my hope is that we can find ways to engage the pharmaceutical companies as allies in our work. I'd like to see the industry reinvent itself as a champion of prevention therapies and cures for early disease, rather than a provider of astronomically expensive last-resort treatment. By channeling their vast resources for research into effective vaccines, better tools for early detection, strategies to protect and bolster the immune system, therapeutics to thwart uncontrolled cell growth, and much more, the industry may be able to find new ways to generate impressive profits.

I asked Otis Brawley, MD, chief medical officer of the American Cancer Society, how pharmaceutical companies would respond if they thought it would be in their best interest to prevent cancer, rather than to treat it. He answered without hesitating: "These companies would jump on it very quickly."

Ultimately, we need "an open and honest discussion at the societal level" to decide how public resources will be used to pay for cancer care, says Dr. Hudis.

Without that, we can expect to continue the cycle that begins when a novel cancer drug wins approval and is put on the market at a very high price, generally accompanied by excitement suggesting it represents a possible breakthrough. Over time, the drug's limitations become apparent, the price drops, competition develops, generic alternatives become available, and the cycle begins again with another new drug.

Meanwhile, our continuing emphasis on producing, prescribing, and paying for one marginally useful cancer therapy after another suggests that we are in the wrong playing field. It tells us we still don't have a winning strategy in the fight against cancer. We can tinker with social policies to help control the cost of cancer drugs—but we're up against a uniquely American resistance to using costs as a factor in our decision making. Our flawed system cries out for reform.

Georgetown University Hospital's Dr. John Marshall thinks the first step toward overhauling the system is to curb the finger pointing. "We often 'demonize' one another," he says, describing the rhetoric as "the drug companies are too greedy; the FDA is too slow; doctors are rich and 'raking it in.'"

To help turn that around, he organized "Fighting a Smarter War against Cancer: Linking Policy to the Patient," a three-day symposium in Washington, DC, in December 2011. The idea was to bring together insurance and pharmaceutical company representatives, government officials, advocates, bioethicists, and others to talk about the concept of value in cancer care. It's a meaningful step toward coming to grips with the many interrelated societal factors that have allowed high-cost, low-benefit therapies to remain dominant.

Still, much more needs to happen to shift our thinking. Until then, people who have been diagnosed with cancer will remain extremely vulnerable. Most don't have the luxury of shopping around for the therapeutic option that offers the greatest benefit at the lowest cost. If a physician advises a specific treatment, few are prepared to question that recommendation. Not many patients have the knowledge or emotional objectivity to dig into the research journals looking for cost-effectiveness analyses and outcome data. Even those who can do that will likely discover that most data are not clear-cut.

Patients are left instead to put their trust in the hands of the medical system—hoping that after all those decades of research and those billions of dollars spent, it can offer an optimal combination of therapies to extend their lives and limit debilitating side effects, without squandering their own, or society's, resources.

Unfortunately, I don't think that's the system we have. Together, we will have to create a better system.

CHAPTER 8

SHIFTING THE RESEARCH APPROACH

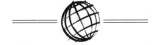

TAKING ON THE MANY WEAKNESSES OF OUR current approach to cancer requires two broad commitments. First, our research focus has to shift from treatment to prevention. "We need to take a fundamental look at our priorities," emphasizes Nirav Shah, MD, MPH, the New York state commissioner of health. "Our priorities do not match our needs. The focus and money is on therapy, rather than prevention."

Second, we need to look hard at the flaws in our existing research infrastructure. Otherwise, we'll be using broken tools to build a new model. It doesn't make a lot of sense to take the system we have now and simply redefine its agenda. From how we describe the mission to how we collect data, conduct clinical trials, and motivate researchers, it is imperative that we approach the cancer challenge in new ways.

NEGLECTING PREVENTION: AN AMERICAN TRADITION

When I asked experts why we haven't focused more on cancer prevention, they emphasized how difficult that kind of research is and how much time it involves. I heard this over and over again, and it disappointed me every time. Had we dedicated just a fraction of all the money we have spent on basic science and marginal treatments for so many years to prevention, we would surely be a lot closer to meeting our goals. We can't continue to squander more time with the unacceptable excuse that the studies are hard to do.

This is a familiar problem, in keeping with a long practice in the United States. We spend huge sums of money on disease, but we don't aggressively implement the prevention tools we already have, nor do we think strategically about how to find new ones.

That will probably startle many Americans, who tend to assume we have the world's healthiest population and the finest-quality care. Certainly, we spend enormous amounts of money on health care. According to the Centers for Medicare and Medicaid Services, $2.6 trillion, or almost 18 percent of the gross domestic product, went toward health care in 2010. Those figures will keep growing, with future costs outpacing the growth of the overall economy. Projections show that by 2020, national health spending will reach $4.6 trillion—almost 20 percent of GDP.[1]

Yet the health status of Americans simply isn't all that good. Despite our optimistic belief in the superiority of our health system, life expectancy in the United States—75.6 years for men, 80.8 years for women—ranks 37th in the world.[2] Geographic, socioeconomic, and racial disparities are pervasive, with the worst health indicators predictably found among less advantaged populations.

There are many reasons for these disparities, including access to health insurance and health services, and the quality of available care, and analysts disagree about what matters most. In our approach to cancer, as with our approach to many other chronic diseases, notably diabetes, we simply do not apply the strategies and practices necessary to save lives.

If we address four major preventable risk factors for disease—smoking, high blood pressure, elevated blood sugar levels, and over-weight—we could increase the life expectancy of men by 4.9 years and women by 4.1 years. We know that raising taxes on tobacco and alcohol, making healthy foods and opportunities for physical activity more readily available, and offering incentives to health insurers and employers to motivate health-promoting behaviors can help decrease these risk factors. Unfortunately, the statistics tell us that we don't use the tools of public health in the service of prevention as much as we should.

Although the National Cancer Institute (NCI) recognizes the power of prevention, calling it "the first line of defense against cancer," its resource allocations clearly emphasize treatment. The NCI's 2012 budget request for its Cancer Prevention and Control program is $232 million. By contrast, its funding request to develop treatments is almost $1.3 billion, or 460 percent more funding.[3]

If the NCI accepts the wisdom and effectiveness of cancer prevention, why isn't it dedicating more resources to it?

The NCI's dominant interest in cancer treatment sets the tone for scientific activities throughout the field. Careers are made from elegant studies of genetics and the cellular mechanisms of cancer, but lives are also saved with behavioral changes, vaccines, and perhaps immunotherapy, which stimulates the body's own immune system to fight cancer.

The President's Cancer Panel, which monitors the nation's cancer program, held a series of meetings in 2010 and 2011 framed around the theme "The Future of Cancer Research: Accelerating Scientific Information." "Areas that are currently inadequately addressed include cancer prevention and early detection," stated panel members in a meeting report. "A shift in strategy is needed to identify informative markers for early detection of cancer; the current approach of analyzing late-stage tumors is unlikely to yield promising leads."[4]

We cannot, of course, turn our backs on those who have already been diagnosed with cancer. Because it will take time to truly change the cancer culture, we need to keep up the hunt for treatments that inhibit the progression of disease. We have the intellectual resources and the capital to pursue *both* agendas, and my intention is *not* to set up prevention in opposition to treatment.

Still, the real work in science and health has to move toward a cancer-free world. That's what our leaders should be talking about, rather than touting the "cancer as a chronic disease" framework as a desirable outcome.

The message should be conveyed at the highest levels. In the White House and in the halls of Congress, our elected officials should be summoning the heads of the nation's preeminent scientific agencies to ask what they are doing to prevent cancer. The finest minds at the National Institutes of Health, the NCI, and elsewhere should come together to redefine the research goal clearly and specifically: Success is the eradication of cancer. Then, they should design a strategy for concentrating our vast and scattered scientific resources to realize that mission. I offer my own vision for a new cancer prevention effort in the next chapter.

Resources are needed for large prevention-focused clinical trials, which often have to run for a decade or more before they can produce results. "They are very, very expensive," says Carolyn R. Aldigé, the founder and president of the nonprofit Prevent Cancer Foundation. "The government has to lead. No one has as much money to fund research as the government."

There is a new reason to expect more results from research dedicated to prevention. Scientists now have cutting-edge ways to study the activity of genes in human tumor samples. More human tissue banks could provide important information about the nature of human cancers and the opportunities to prevent them.

Recasting the current, scattershot approach to studying cancer into a laser-focused quest to prevent it is only one component of the shift we need. Another is recognizing and correcting the terrible flaws in our current research enterprise, in which there is a drive for personal gain, a duplication of efforts, conflicts of interests, and so little oversight that outright fraud is possible. The American people deserve better than that.

ABSENT TEAM SCIENCE

Too many of the resources dedicated to fighting cancer are used to establish new programs, branches, panels, subdivisions, and agencies. Without a more consolidated effort, no one has the authority to set the agenda and then chart the course for achieving it. The result is a fragmented, repetitive approach in which too much money is spent on buildings and bureaucracy and too many researchers work in isolation.

Within the federal government, cancer programs are lodged at the Department of Health and Human Services, the Department of Energy, the Department of Defense, and the Environmental Protection Agency. In addition to the sprawling NCI, which is accountable directly to the president, Health and Human Services serves as an umbrella for cancer work at the Agency for Healthcare Research and Quality, the Centers for Disease Control and Prevention, the FDA, the Health Resources and Service Administration, and the National Institutes of Health. There is a lack of coordination, too much overlap, and too few opportunities for one entity to learn what the other is doing. Precious time and resources are being lost.

Scientists should be sharing information, thinking about how their work complements that of their colleagues, and looking for opportunities to engage people in other disciplines to bring added value to their research. Instead, they often work in distant silos, competing for the same funds and protecting their data fiercely. Their futures depend on publishing their findings in prestigious journals or making patentable discoveries with the potential for great profits, not on sharing data. There are, of course, professional meetings where researchers gather and share ideas, but this offers only a limited opportunity for exchanging data.

The NCI does have programs to promote collaboration, but these are too often inefficiently designed, and the applications required for participation can be burdensome. There is too much "what's in it for me?" and not enough "we're all in this together."

The result, wrote Sharon Begley in *Newsweek*, is "a lot of elegant science and important research papers," but not much advancement in patient care. In a grim analysis, aptly titled "We Fought Cancer . . . and Cancer Won," she said, "It is possible (and common) for cancer researchers to achieve extraordinary acclaim and success, measured by grants, awards, professorships and papers in leading journals, without ever helping a single patient gain a single extra day of life. There is no pressure within science to make that happen."[5]

This self-centered attitude is not the one that took us to the moon. The National Aeronautics and Space Agency's (NASA) signature approach had been to set a specific goal and a specific deadline for accomplishing it—in this case, landing a man on the moon in the next 10 years. With the objective defined, NASA applied a model of collaboration designed to converge on the bull's-eye. Dr. Ronald Herberman was there in the 1970s when the NCI invited experts from NASA to explain their organizational strategies.

Dr. Herberman recalls the diagrams the space agency used to illustrate its framework. "There were a series of concentric circles where the initial steps in the process and the planning stages were in the outermost circles. Once everything is accomplished in the outer circles, you progress inward until you get to the center." For NASA, the centerpiece was the walk on the moon; for NCI, it should have been the cure for cancer.

NCI officials did not embrace the idea, feeling that cancer was too complex to address with a single goal. Rather than adopting NASA's convergent approach, it chose a divergent model, with the idea that allowing many researchers to follow many competing paths would be the best way to move forward.

The limits of that approach are now evident to me and to many of the experts with whom I have been speaking.

FAILED DATA MANAGEMENT

Collecting and sharing data is one of the most important tools for advancing research, yet our current system is "unbelievably inefficient," according to Laura Esserman, MD, who directs the Carol Franc Buck Breast Care Center at the University of California, San Francisco.[6]

Good data is the foundation of almost everything we do in cancer care, and everything we need to do to achieve the goal of prevention. Effective data management allows us to learn about and build on clinical and research experiences across the vast cancer field. It sheds light on who has responded best to what kind of treatment, and allows us to offer optimal health services to patients who receive care at more than one location. Sharing data across clinical trials also adds power to studies that may have enrolled a limited population or lasted for a relatively short period of time.

Consider the importance of good data in personalized medicine, a fledgling discipline that many of us believe holds tremendous promise for tailoring prevention or treatment to the individual characteristics of the patient or the tumor.

Personalized medicine contrasts with the "homogenous, one-glove-fits-all" approach that we tend to use now, points out Thomas Degnan, MD, who is retired as co-chief of the Don Monti Division of Hematology and Oncology and chairman of the department of research at the North Shore University Hospital in Manhasset, New

York. Yet cancer itself is anything but homogenous. There are vast differences in how it lodges, reproduces, and spreads within and outside of its place of origin. Treatments that are effective in one subset of the population may harm another.

"In any given individual, cancer imparts a distinctive signature extending from molecular presentation to response to treatment and overall survival," Dr. Degnan says. We believe that when we can read that signature, we will be much better able to personalize our approach by custom-tailoring the timing and nature of the intervention. The key to doing that is to be able to collect and analyze biomarkers, the biological indicators of a disease state, and to understand what they predict about the need for treatment and the timing for administering it. "Interventions could occur before disease appears," he explains.

Efficient data systems are essential to that kind of knowledge across research settings. The authors of an article in *Clinical Cancer Research* described the need clearly: "By creating information networks that follow patients longitudinally over time, and identifying patients who share both clinical characteristics and unique molecular cancer biomarkers, researchers and clinicians may be able to predict clinical outcomes and determine the value of certain diagnostics or interventions for specific patient populations."[7]

To put it simply, a well-managed information system "will be the basis for providing the right treatment for the right patient in the right place at the right time," they wrote.

Beyond the immediate patient benefits, improving data collection encourages team science. Everyone has to share the responsibility of feeding the system, and everyone has to have access to the knowledge it provides. That means primary care physicians, public and private insurance companies, investigators conducting clinical trials, and epidemiologists collecting surveillance data should all be able to contribute data, stripped of information that allows that data to be traced to specific patients. Each of these players should then be able to use the data to guide his or her own treatment approaches and research activities, as should community medical centers, primary care clinics, specialty cancer hospitals, research institutions, government scientists, and others.

We are far from being able to do most of this. Indeed, a 2008 survey found that only 1.5 percent of the participating 3,049 acute-care hospitals had established a comprehensive system for maintaining electronic medical records. An additional 7.6 percent of responding hospitals had a minimal system in place, defined as electronic records in at least one clinical unit.[8]

Significant change is needed before electronic health records can be put into widespread use. In addition to the need for financial support, we have to train adequate numbers of information technology experts to build functional systems. Even more daunting is creating interoperability—the capacity of different electronic systems to share and exchange data. If a single hospital can't even share data across departments, imagine how far we are from systems that can gather information from thousands and thousands of sites.

While it is troubling that electronic data management lags significantly within hospitals and among individual clinicians, the absence of an effective information system at the NCI is astounding.

NCI's Cancer Biomedical Informatics Grid (caBIG), launched in 2004, was an attempt to change that. One of the NCI's most far-reaching programs, CaBIG sought to connect the entire cancer community, from bench scientists to cancer clinicians to the FDA, by creating a next-generation collaborative infrastructure for biomedical research.[9]

At the time, as now, there was no single system allowing cancer researchers to exchange information. A cancer center in California experimenting with a new chemotherapy had no way of knowing whether a cancer center in Maine had already demonstrated good results using the same drug. The hope was to integrate information from studies that looked at related questions from different perspectives—for example, aggregating the analyses of multiple researchers who are each looking at a single step in the process that allows a tumor to take root or analyzing the reasons why a cancer cell eventually stops responding to therapy.

CaBIG was supposed to make that possible, and by allowing data to be readily shared, it was also supposed to accelerate scientific discoveries. It was built on grid technology, which Andrea Califano, PhD, who is the founding director and chair of the Genome Center at Columbia University's medical center, describes as a way "to take a computational program and distribute it over the Internet to computers that may be unknown to you." Califano, who was head of the working group within the NCI's Board of Scientific Advisors assigned to review caBIG, likens the system to Apple's iCloud. With cloud computing, a user takes a photo, uploads it to the cloud—which could be a computer anywhere in the world—and retrieves it at will. While the computer's exact location is irrelevant to the scientists who use it, only the capacity to access the data it contains is essential.

The striking feature of caBIG is that it offered the opportunity to collect, integrate, analyze, and disseminate vast stores of information. With research projects under way that involve thousands of DNA sequences and proteins, that kind of technology does more than reduce the arduous analytical processes involved in studying the behavior of cancer; it makes it possible. "If you tried to figure out the combinations manually, the numbers would be so spectacularly large that it would not be feasible," Califano says.

Despite the ambition and the hope, caBIG veered off course. Seven years and $350 million after its launch, the NCI imposed a one-year moratorium on the project.

In March 2011, the Board of Scientific Advisors working group issued a report concluding that caBIG had expanded far beyond its original goals "to implement an overly complex and ambitious software enterprise." The report said tools produced through caBIG had "limited traction in the cancer community, compete against established commercial vendors and create financially untenable long-term maintenance and support commitments for the NCI."[10]

Califano was even more explicit when we spoke. CaBIG, he says, was powerful, far-reaching technology, but developers lacked a clear understanding of how it would be used. "It was a clear case of putting the cart before the horse. Instead of having biological problems define the technology, we had technology developed, waiting for problems to come up."

Fundamental flaws included a lack of independent external oversight and funding decisions that did not incorporate a system of peer review—the people who would actually use the information were not adequately consulted. "It was never demonstrated that this new technology would help cancer researchers do their job," Califano says. The grid technology proved to complicate, rather than enhance, the core goal of allowing researchers to share data. Huge sums were spent on external consultants, who lacked expertise in basic or clinical science. In addition, a lack of transparency in awarding software development contracts permitted conflicts of interest. Complex layers of management and the use of expensive consultants created a barrier between the research community and caBIG's leadership.

In December 2011, caBIG's director resigned, and the NCI announced plans to overhaul the entire initiative. The concept of enhancing the exchange and integration of data remains sound, and some of the tools necessary to make that happen continue to be developed. However, we are still a long way from realizing the goals caBIG first articulated almost a decade ago, and the lack of an adequate information infrastructure continues to hinder efforts to build knowledge. Califano bemoans that fact, commenting, "In cancer, we are trying to build a 747 with an abacus."

FLAWED CLINICAL TRIAL DESIGN

Good medicine is built on clinical trials in which promising scientific discoveries are tested in human beings. The National Cancer Institute guides the nation's largest trial network, principally through its Clinical Trials Cooperative Group Program. Its 24,000 investigators at more than 3,100 institutions enroll some 25,000 patients every year.

This essential element of the cancer infrastructure is also in dire need of a broad restructuring. A 2010 Institute of Medicine (IOM) report stated that the current framework "is approaching a state of crisis. . . . If the clinical trials system does not improve its efficiency and effectiveness, the introduction of new treatments for cancer will be delayed and patient lives will be lost unnecessarily."[11] It also emphasized that across-the-board changes are urgently needed.

One of the weaknesses cited by the IOM is a "lengthy and redundant process" for designing, reviewing, and initiating clinical trials, which allows years to elapse after an idea is conceived and before the first patient is enrolled. No adequate mechanisms are in place for establishing priorities, so there is no way to ensure that the most promising trials proceed the most quickly. Long delays can also make it more difficult to recruit patients into research studies. Ultimately, only about 60 percent of the NCI-supported trials complete the journey from launch to published results, "a terrible waste of human and financial resources," according to the report.

Inadequate NCI funding for clinical trials is another problem. This invariably forces investigators to seek supplementary funds from pharmaceutical companies and other sources, which creates an inherent bias and raises the specter of conflict of interest. In addition, physicians may not have incentives for enrolling their patients in clinical trials, and patients often incur associated costs that are not reimbursed by insurance providers.

To transform a system that it called "inefficient and cumbersome," the IOM recommended consolidating functions within the clinical trial network, enhancing collaboration and funding, establishing priorities, and speeding up the trial process from start to finish. It also called for developing novel approaches and new technologies to "incorporate innovative science and trial design" and for recruiting larger, more diverse populations into trials more quickly and covering the cost of their care. "Collectively, implementation of the recommendations presented in this report will lead to the faster approval and adoption of new therapies, new discoveries upon which to base future studies, and the accelerated translation of new knowledge into beneficial therapies for patients with cancer."

Let's hope so. Whether the NCI will truly transform its entire system of clinical trials remains to be seen, but the oncology field does seem to be taking the recommendations seriously. A year after the report, the American Society of Clinical Oncology sponsored a workshop in partnership with the IOM to review the NCI's progress in detail, and that kind of critique is scheduled to happen again.[12] Professional societies and government leaders should endorse the IOM's recommendations and continue to watch closely to make sure they are implemented.

———

Too often, clinical trials fail to discover who will benefit from a therapy and who will be harmed. Yet the highly acclaimed promise of personalized medicine depends on this knowledge. If we aren't extracting it from our studies, we can wind up approving drugs without knowing who should actually be using them.

We saw what can happen as a result after the FDA licensed the monoclonal antibody cetuximab in 2004 to treat advanced colorectal cancer. The drug provides its very short survival benefit by binding to a protein that is overexpressed in many human cancers, an action intended to curb the growth of the cancer cells. After cetuximab was approved, researchers discovered that the drug can be harmful to patients who have a particular genetic mutation known as K-ras. That includes about 40 percent of patients with metastatic colorectal cancer.

Five years after cetuximab reached the market, the American Society for Clinical Oncology advised that doctors test all patients with metastatic colorectal cancer for the K-ras mutation—and to avoid prescribing any drug in the same class to those who have it.[13]

By then, some 100,000 patients with the mutation had "received unhelpful and potentially detrimental therapy," according to an analysis published in *Clinical Cancer Research*.[14]

"We need to recognize that not all colorectal cancers are the same," says Georgetown University Hospital's Dr. John Marshall. He could be talking about any other cancer in the body when he adds, "We need to place our effort on not just cranking people through empiric therapies, but deciding which empiric therapies are working for which patients."

Likewise, we need to be doing the studies that will tell us which colon cancer patients require chemotherapy. Dr. Marshall says that surgery cures at least 75 percent of patients with stage II colon cancer. Of the remaining 25 percent who are not cured by surgery, only 3 to 5 percent will actually see added benefit from chemotherapy. Because we don't know the profile of those who will gain, almost all patients routinely get chemotherapy. That translates into "giving therapies that fail 95 percent of the time in order to find that 3 to 5 percent of responsive patients," he says.

Creating a tumor bank to which physicians routinely send samples of all stage II colon cancers would eventually generate the molecular profiles necessary to enable these critical distinctions. Making that happen, however, involves grappling with another complexity of the system: patient privacy laws, which currently hinder the sharing of medical data.

Even devoid of personally identifiable information, the federal Health Insurance Portability and Accountability Act (HIPAA) requires every patient to give permission before any information about his or her disease can be released.

This cumbersome process has made it harder to aggregate knowledge and means that many important studies either are not conducted at all or are done using data collected in other countries. "HIPAA is a terrible law from a research perspective," Dr. Marshall says. "I understand the need for privacy, but we should be clever enough to overcome the obstacles." One way to do that is an act of Congress that would allow any patient data obtained in a federally funded trial to be included, anonymously, in a database.

RESEARCH FRAUD

Every cancer has a distinctive genetic pattern. If we can identify the DNA sequences that characterize a patient's particular cancer, we will have, in essence, a next-generation biomarker. The hope is that we can figure out which drug works best for a cancer with a particular genomic signature.

In 2006, researchers at Duke University claimed to have done just that, and numerous prestigious medical journals published their analysis, including *Lancet Oncology,* the *Journal of Clinical Oncology, Nature Medicine,* and the *New England Journal of Medicine.* "We developed gene expression signatures that predict sensitivity to individual chemotherapeutic drugs. . . . We further show that many of these signatures can accurately predict clinical response," the researchers announced in *Nature Medicine.*[15]

The team, led by Anil Potti, MD, an oncologist and assistant professor of medicine at Duke, maintained that its data could be used to develop tests that matched patients who had breast, ovarian, and other cancers to appropriate therapies. Based on their research, the National Cancer Institute funded three large clinical trials. The authors also became involved in CancerGuide Diagnostics, a start-up company intent on commercializing the use of genomic signatures. Duke University joined them in claiming an equity interest in the company.

All that was based on a fraudulent manipulation of data.

The falsified medical research began to unravel when Keith A. Baggerly, PhD, a biostatistician at MD Anderson Cancer Center, and his colleague, Kevin R. Coombes, PhD, tried to replicate the findings. When their own analysis could not lead them to the same genomic signatures and their review of the Duke data revealed other errors, they asked Dr. Potti's research team for an explanation but were rebuffed. Baggerly and Coombes then reported their concerns to Duke's Institutional Review Board, which is charged with ensuring the ethical conduct of clinical trials. Ultimately, they spoke out publicly and described some of the missteps that were putting patients at risk. "Poor documentation can shift from an inconvenience to an active danger when it obscures not just methods, but errors," they wrote in the *Annals of Applied Statistics*.[16]

Few people listened closely. Only when Paul Goldberg, the editor and publisher of the *Cancer Letter*, uncovered a bit of false information on Dr. Potti's résumé—he had claimed to be a Rhodes scholar but was not—did the scientific community finally take action. In July 2010, 31 scientists called on the National Cancer Institute to suspend the trials at Duke, and the NCI finally did so. Dr. Potti was placed on paid administrative leave, and the American Cancer Society suspended a $729,000 grant it had given him.[17]

Retractions of the published research began in 2010, with an article that had appeared in the *Journal of Clinical Oncology*. By February 2012, the authors had issued retractions in eight more peer-reviewed journals, and others were expected. Some of these articles had been cited hundreds of times by researchers.[18]

As the extent of the deception came to light, investigations began. The NCI asked the Institute of Medicine to examine the Duke scandal and to recommend best practices to guide the development of "omics-based" tests in the future. Omics includes genomics, the study of the DNA sequences of an organism, and proteomics, the large-scale study of proteins. In its report, the IOM laid out a set of procedures to improve the pathway from discovery to the first use of an omics-based test in clinical trials, including new approaches to recording, validating, and protecting data and ensuring adequate oversight.[19]

More dramatically, the IOM report stated that the systems in place "to ensure the integrity and rigor of the scientific process failed" and made clear that Duke was not unique in allowing that to occur. The systemic breakdown included "the failure of scientific collaboration, review processes by journals, regulatory oversight, institutional systems for protection of patient-participants and institutional systems for management of conflicts of interest."

People with cancer were the real losers. Some who had enrolled in clinical trials based on the Duke research "lost the chance to enroll in another trial that might have had real benefit," says Keith Baggerly. Others might have been harmed by the biopsies required to participate in the studies. "A lung biopsy in a patient with advanced disease can render the patient unstable enough to be unable to participate in standard-of-care chemotherapy. If this is part of a legitimate trial, and there is informed consent, that's acceptable. If the investigators know that the clinical trial is based on 'garbage data,' then it is unethical," he adds.

Dr. Potti has since resigned, and a lawsuit has been filed against Duke on behalf of eight patients who charge that university officials "breached their ethical, moral, and 'responsible party' duties."[20] As the legal repercussions play out, the public trust in science, medicine, and the safety of participating in research trials has been dealt a hard blow.

That sloppy science, flagrant conflicts of interest, and outright deceit could escape detection at a prestigious academic center and the nation's finest medical journals should underscore the urgent need for change.

Much stricter guidelines are needed to ensure adequate data management, rigorous team science, and systems of accountability, and they need to be much more rigorously enforced. Without adequate oversight, we cannot meet our most fundamental obligation to protect patients.

CONFLICTS OF INTEREST

There is a great deal of money to be made in scientific discovery. Two high-profile cases illustrate how conflicts of interest can result and how they can endanger unbiased, patient-centered research.

One case involves Craig Thompson, MD, the president and CEO of Memorial Sloan-Kettering Cancer Center. As reported in the *New York Times*, Thompson has been sued by his former employer, the Leonard and Madlyn Abramson Family Cancer Research Institute at the University of Pennsylvania (Penn), for laying claim to intellectual property and building his own business on it. Separately, Penn has filed its own lawsuit.[21]

At the heart of the dispute are questions about who owns the fruits of scientific research and the patents that follow from it. In 2007, Thompson launched a biotechnology company called Agios, which filed for patents on some of the cancer metabolism research conducted at Penn that had been designed to examine metabolic changes in cancer cells. The resulting clash stemmed from the common expectation that universities will be able to control the inventions made on their campuses, and the revenues that flow from them.

The twists and turns of the story will be ironed out through the legal system, but huge sums of money are at stake: Penn claims $100 million in damages while the Abramson lawsuit puts its potential damages at $1 billion. The language of the Abramson action is particularly blunt: Dr. Thompson "chose to abscond with the fruits of the Abramson largesse generated by his work at the Institute and thereby cheat future generations of the intended benefits of the donation and the Institute's intellectual property."[22] This case represents, at the very least, an unnecessary misunderstanding and a waste of precious time and resources.

A similar case involved a successful cancer treatment built on technology developed at the University of Alabama by J. Milton Harris, PhD, Distinguished Professor of Chemistry. Here, too, the dispute centered on patents that earned substantial revenue for industry but cut the university out of profits generated by faculty research. The university settled the litigation in 2006 for $25 million.[23]

The earlier story of the Duke fraud and these two conflicts between researchers and their academic employers are examples of how the pursuit of private profit has the potential to undermine the real humanitarian calling of science. The agenda of what has come to be known as "the cancer enterprise" also colors the commitment to putting the best interests of patients first. There are certainly important benefits of having scientists collaborate with the drug industry, which has the capacity to commercialize research findings and get them to patients. However, safeguards are necessary to avoid the significant risks.

In a "Perspectives" article in the *New England Journal of Medicine,* Bernard Lo, MD, of the University of California, San Francisco, highlighted the different missions of academic health centers and pharmaceutical companies.[24] In theory, he wrote, one seeks "to understand the mechanisms of disease and human functioning," while the other aims to "develop new products that will generate profits for the company." One aims to "promote evidence-based medicine and independent critical judgment by physicians" while the other's intention is "to develop marketing strategies to improve sales and profits."

Academic scientists sometimes have a foot in both camps, hoping to add to the storehouse of knowledge and clinical options for patients while also gaining financial benefit. They do this not only by starting companies to commercialize their findings but also by serving on corporate boards in their fields, where they are often paid generously for their service. None of this is inherently unethical, but careful conflict-of-interest policies are needed to guide these activities and to ensure that the desire to make money does not skew scientific judgment. Many institutions haven't enacted such policies.

After carefully observing the many places where conflicts of interest can occur, the Institute of Medicine offered detailed recommendations about how best to avoid them. Its report, *Conflict of Interest in Medical Research, Education and Practice,* emphasized that merely disclosing conflicts is not enough, calling it "a critical but limited first step."[25] Among other strategies, the IOM urged that industry be required to make any payments to researchers public information and that researchers not be permitted to conduct studies if they have a financial interest in the outcome (for example, because they hold a patent on a therapy).

Good science, not great profit, needs to drive medicine, or else no one will have confidence in the system. As the IOM report stated, "Patients and the public need to be able to trust that the high costs of health care and health insurance arise from the provision of services that are beneficial, necessary, appropriately priced, and not inappropriately driven by the financial interests of physicians, other health care providers or medical product companies."

Fixing the System

The challenge of overhauling the system may seem daunting, yet I remain optimistic that we can be nimble enough to take on cancer in new ways. Progress demands an emphasis on collaborative research that is designed, funded, and implemented with adherence to rigorous guidelines that target the goal of eradicating cancer.

If we are to succeed, we must have firm, focused leaders to redefine our goal as preventing cancer, and the political will to dedicate the resources and build the infrastructure necessary to accomplish that mission. Scientists in government, academia, and industry must cease their isolated pursuit of knowledge and collaborate in a meaningful exchange of data.

Today, one researcher may be studying a mutation in the cellular DNA, another looking at a chromosomal abnormality, and a third scrutinizing the way a gene expresses itself. These threads of information need to be stitched together.

"Right now, we look at one thing at a time," says Andrea Califano of Columbia University's Genome Center. "Unfortunately, the tumor couldn't care less. It's a fully integrated complex of problems."

If the problems are integrated, the solutions must be as well. "In other disciplines, collaboration is the modus operandi," he emphasizes. "We cannot do systems biology without combining computational biology, molecular biology, engineering, and many other fields. Papers in systems biology are written by multiple authors with a great amount of collaboration. A paper would not be written without that collaboration."

For example, an interdisciplinary group of physicists, scientists, engineers, mathematicians, and others are developing an 18-mile supercollider, which Califano describes as "four times the length of a Washington, DC, Metro tunnel," to study the most fundamental particles of the universe. If we can dedicate that kind of commitment to understanding the laws of nature, we should be doing no less than engaging the world's finest scientific minds to prevent cancer.

There are other examples of how effective team science can be. The Cystic Fibrosis Foundation has built a research model that has demonstrated its value with results. Although the disease still cannot be cured, treatments are now available that effectively double the life span of patients with the disease—young people who might once have died in their 20s now routinely live into their 40s. That happened through "managed, strategic approaches," according to Marc Hurlbert, PhD, the executive director of breast cancer programs of the Avon Foundation for Women and the Avon Breast Cancer Crusade. Molecular biologists, immunologists, medicinal chemists, and others worked together to tackle the disease.

The National Cancer Institute should be doing much the same thing. "I'm not saying blow up the NCI," Hurlbert emphasizes. "Rather, the NCI should bring in new strategies and project managers and encourage scientists to focus on specific goals that would include the causes and prevention of cancer."

Without further delay, we should harness the talent and resources already at work on cancer in new ways, drawing on 21st-century information systems built to allow the easy exchange of data. Above all, we need our scientific pioneers to work together, with funding and other incentives aligned to encourage that. Career success, and the promotions that come with it, must be defined by allegiance to team science, not personal ambition. Califano is insistent about that, saying, "We need to abrogate the boundaries built by the need to be competitive against each other as cancer researchers."

CHAPTER 9

THE PROMISE OF PREVENTION

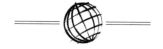

THERE IS MUCH WE CAN DO TODAY TO FORE-
stall cancer, making the absence of urgency outrageous.
"We know now what behaviors can reduce cancer risk,"
says Prevent Cancer's Carolyn R. Aldigé. "If we applied what we
know right now, we could reduce cancer by 50 percent."

Researcher Graham Colditz, MD, DrPH, agreed. After evaluat-
ing the impact of "research-proven strategies and interventions," he
concluded that more than half of all cancers need not occur.[1] Dr.
Colditz is director of prevention and control at the Alvin J. Siteman
Cancer Center and a professor at Washington University School of
Medicine.

If it is true that results from prevention research can take decades,

I say let's not waste any more time. Long-term prevention studies launched 20 years ago would have given us crucial answers today, and many people might never have suffered with cancer.

"Doctors are trying to deal with what's broken already, rather than trying to prevent it from getting broken," says Robert P. Heaney, MD, a professor of medicine at John A. Creighton University School of Medicine in Omaha.

To realign our approach, I propose that we create a bold new initiative: the National Cancer Prevention Institute (NCPI). This entity, built as part of the National Institutes of Health (NIH) to target cancer prevention exclusively, would coordinate the many cloistered activities throughout the federal government and lead the way into new arenas.

Where will the money come from? In these challenging economic times, when federal and state budgets are being reduced, this is a legitimate question. Ideally, Congress would provide new funding for the NCPI, based on the pressing needs it will address and the fact that a dedicated cancer prevention strategy saves money in the long run.

If those revenues are not forthcoming, we will have to reallocate resources from the many line items in the federal budget currently dedicated to cancer. By drawing from the existing budgets of the NIH, the National Cancer Institute (NCI), and other federal cancer initiatives, proportional to their size, the NCPI need not add to the overall resource burden.

It is not as if the NIH isn't already funding new health research programs. It is just that the design of those programs is as flawed as the current ones.

In 2012, the NIH established the National Center for Advancing Translational Science (NCATS), reallocating funds from its other programs to generate a $639 million budget. NCATS is supposed to accelerate the pace of research so that drugs, vaccines, and diagnostic tests will become available to patients sooner. It is not actually charged with developing new therapies, but rather with finding innovative ways to push out scientific discoveries more quickly.

Separately, the NIH launched the Cures Acceleration Network (CAN), with $10 million in start-up funding in 2012, and a request for an additional $39.6 million in 2013. Its purpose is "to accelerate the development of high need cures by reducing barriers between research discovery and clinical trials."[2]

Neither NCATS nor CAN will exclusively target cancer, and frankly, there appears to be considerable overlap in their goals. Both continue the federal government's fractured approach, giving short shrift to prevention. NCATS has already established partnerships with the pharmaceutical industry to study drugs that failed to treat the medical conditions for which they were originally designed but that might be useful in other ways. All of that suggests to me that the federal government will spend more money and the pharmaceutical industry will earn more profits, but that people with cancer will continue to die.

How the National Cancer Prevention Institute Will Be Different

The launch of the NCPI is designed to make cancer prevention a national priority. Most of its work should be built around applied epidemiology—studies of how and why diseases are distributed across populations and how those diseases can be controlled. It will help us understand what the differences are between people with cancer and without it while seeking meaningful tools of early detection; how vaccines prevent cancer or send it into enduring remission; and what roles nutritional deficiencies, environmental exposures, and genetic risk factors play in the disease.

As I envision it, the NCPI will set focused and specific goals and attach deadlines to them. Each team of researchers and scientists in each division will oversee a particular cancer—such as brain, breast, colon, lung, ovarian, pancreatic, prostate, as well as leukemia, lymphoma, and other cancers—with a commitment to reducing its incidence by a certain percentage during a particular time frame. Organ-specific cancer prevention research will be fully integrated across divisions; resources, data, and discoveries will be shared openly. With cancer prevention as the ultimate goal, a victory for one type of cancer will be a victory for all.

Each division will allocate about 90 percent of its budget for research, funding work on specific cancers in universities and cancer centers across the country. The remaining 10 percent will be spent on intramural research conducted by staff scientists within the institute, and on management of each division. The opportunities for epidemiological research are many—for example, nutritional deficiencies, exposures to environmental chemicals, and the presence of viruses can be compared in healthy people and those with cancer.

Each year, the NCPI will update Congress on its progress. All stakeholders—representatives from government, the pharmaceutical industry, health insurance companies, patient advocates, physicians, and scientists—will help to shape its agenda, and they will be asked to contribute their resources and knowledge to its mission. Specialists in epidemiology, microbiology, systems biology, engineering, oncology, immunology, pharmaceuticals, and more will all be involved, recognizing that there is a better chance to prevent cancer through collaboration and true team science.

The NCPI will give us the infrastructure we need to move forward. This core principle will be embedded in its design: Researchers have more to gain from sharing their findings broadly than they do from holding them close for fear of losing some perceived edge. Their rewards will be in discovering effective strategies and agents to prevent cancer and in seeing those measures reduce the incidence of cancer.

"It's about learning to trust each other," emphasizes Columbia University's Andrea Califano. "It's about learning that when you protect your own data to get an extra publication, you're preventing yourself from working with a much more exciting set of data that wouldn't otherwise be available. It takes courageous people to do that, but that's the way biology is going to progress."

Through a system of peer review and targeted funding, the NCPI will empower the scientific community in the United States to lead and inspire a global effort. With a collective commitment from every sector of American society, we will discard what is weak, wasteful, and inept in our current system, maintain and bolster what works, and move on to a new era.

PUBLIC HEALTH: GOVERNMENT AS STEWARD

As the NCPI implements the scientific agenda, government at the federal, state, and local levels should be coordinating a much more aggressive public health effort.

Public health concerns itself with the health of populations, rather than with the care of individual patients. It is about sweeping and often-inexpensive actions that can have very broad impact. Getting people vaccinated, restricting smoking, improving access to fresh fruits and vegetables, and removing contaminants from the environment are all core public health activities. Although these crucial initiatives don't often make headlines, they do save lives.

Two of the nation's most devastating public health problems—the twin epidemics of smoking and obesity—contribute significantly to cancer, and so aggressive public health action here will have a multiplier effect. An analysis in *Science Translational Medicine* tells us that one-third of all cancers in the United States are caused by smoking. Overweight and obesity are responsible for an additional 20 percent of cancer, with diet and lack of exercise each causing another 5 percent.[3] In total, these factors are responsible for more than 50 percent of all cancers.

Yet public health is largely invisible because its primary function is to prevent bad things from happening, rather than to cure them once they do, and so public health has historically been underfunded and underappreciated.

"It is easy for people to take it for granted when, on any particular day, they don't get sick at work (because of air-quality improvements), aren't poisoned (because the food is safe) or don't get run over (because the walkway has been separated from the road)," wrote David Hemenway, PhD, professor of health policy at the Harvard School of Public Health, in the *New England Journal of Medicine*. By contrast, medicine is "flashy, its master practitioners and innovators lionized, and its accomplishments widely celebrated."[4]

Our new assault on cancer will have to bring public health to the center stage.

With government investing its authority and resources in prevention, we can bring a powerhouse of new ideas and talent to the effort. In an era when there is so much resistance to using the tools of government to shape society, I know some will argue that the government has no right to tell people how to behave. Cries of a "nanny state" invariably arise; we saw this in New York City when the health department banned the use of artery-clogging trans fats in restaurants, and we have seen it across the country as municipalities and states imposed bans on smoking in public places.

No doubt we'll hear such protests again as new initiatives are proposed to make it easier for people to avoid tobacco, to eat better, and to exercise. We'll also see industry fighting efforts to ban carcinogenic chemicals, pharmaceutical interests defending their unfettered right to profit from marginally effective drugs, and insurance companies reluctant to add prevention to the stream of services for which they provide reimbursement.

Amid all this noise and resistance, we will have to move steadily forward, recognizing that every sector of society has a role to play in shifting from a focus on treatment to a focus on prevention, and all of us stand to gain. Cancer has a devastating impact not only on the individuals and families who receive a cancer diagnosis but also on a society that simply can't afford the costs. A healthy, vibrant population is key to a healthy, vibrant nation.

In the next several chapters, I offer some specific ideas about how government can advance cancer prevention by encouraging healthier living. Along the way, we will have to bring in 21st-century tools of social marketing and social media to design messages about how individuals can change their own behavior and about what public and private organizations can do to support that change.

We'll need government funding for communication campaigns

that galvanize attention, using public service announcements, high-profile celebrities, viral videos, graphic images, and many other tested approaches to get the word out. The possibilities are limited only by our imagination.

Our young people should be riveted by age-appropriate messages from film, television, and sports stars they admire. These role models should be telling teenagers that it is cool not to smoke, to drink water instead of sweetened soft drinks, to eat an apple rather than a bag of chips, and to get enough physical exercise. Just as television presents brief and moving memorials of soldiers lost in war, so, too, we might try publishing the photographs of people lost to cancer on our social media sites—along with messages about how such tragedies can be averted.

Creativity and evidence of direct impact will have to drive these and other marketing efforts, and messages will likely need to be presented differently to different target populations. "There are both well-educated and poorly educated people who need to change their behavior," emphasizes Prevent Cancer Foundation's Carolyn R. Aldigé. To reach as many Americans as possible, campaigns need to target specific cultural groups, including Spanish speakers, Native Americans, Asian-Americans, and others, as well as populations with varying levels of education and income.

Beyond research and education, the government's role in transforming our whole approach to cancer is intricately tied to some of the larger challenges of the health care system. Collaborative efforts are needed to resolve the complex issues of equity, cost, and insurance reimbursement in order to build the framework we need.

One major issue that government must rigorously address is the tremendous disparities in cancer care. Income, race and ethnicity, insurance status, and geography all influence the ability of an individual to get appropriate screening, timely diagnosis, and adequate treatment. "*Where* you live should not determine *whether* or not you will live," insists Chandini Portteus, vice president for research, evaluation, and scientific programs at Susan G. Komen for the Cure.

Unfortunately, geography and many other demographic characteristics often do have influence. People in certain urban neighborhoods and rural communities have higher rates of cancer. African Americans are more likely to develop cancer than any other racial group, less likely to receive appropriate follow-up for findings suspicious of colon cancer, and less likely to receive radiation after breast cancer surgery. People without insurance are screened less often for certain cancers, wait longer before their cancer is diagnosed, and die more quickly from it. Low-income women are less likely to be prescribed appropriate drugs following a breast cancer diagnosis.[5]

The reasons for these disparities are many and complex. One factor is the way we do research. Most of what we know about the risk and progression of cancer comes from studies that enroll Caucasian populations, according to a President's Cancer Panel report.[6] That means we haven't looked closely at whether there are distinctive characteristics of different racial populations contributing to the unequal cancer burden.

In the same vein, we have not devoted enough attention to what are called the social determinants of health—features like a person's education, access to resources, and conditions of daily life, beginning at birth and extending across the life span. In its report, the President's Cancer Panel emphasized the importance of examining "the complex interplay of numerous socioeconomic, cultural, environmental, biological, behavioral and genetic factors" that influence cancer risk and outcomes.[7] The report outlines specific gaps in what we need to know in order to provide more timely and culturally sensitive care to an increasingly diverse American population.

Along with paying more attention to these issues, the federal government must leverage the vast resources it spends on health care to direct more attention to prevention and cost control. Together, Medicare (the nation's largest insurer of American adults), Medicaid, and the Children's Health Insurance Program cost the federal government $769 billion in 2011, or more than one-fifth of the total budget, according to the Washington-based Center on Budget and Policy Priorities.[8]

Linking reimbursement to care that keeps people healthy, rather than simply paying for more treatment, is essential. The power of that kind of money should also give government a sizable edge in negotiating down the price of cancer drugs. Many federal government strategies set an example for private insurance responses as well, so this all can have an augmented impact.

THE ROLE OF THE MEDICAL COMMUNITY

The medical community must be a dynamic player in efforts to bring prevention forward, both in one-on-one interactions with patients and in the national agenda.

Current reimbursement structures make it difficult for time-pressured physicians to schedule opportunities to talk to their patients about all-important, cancer-preventing lifestyle changes. "Doctors get paid to prescribe and administer treatment," says Dr. Otis Brawley of the American Cancer Society. "Right now, there is a disincentive for doctors to speak with patients about prevention. I'd like to see the system turned upside down. I'd like to see physicians paid for prevention counseling, not treatment. I'd like to see a system more interested in keeping people out of the 'sick care' part of the system."

Until we create the infrastructure that rewards prevention, we will keep relying on the goodwill of individual physicians to make that happen. Like many dedicated practitioners, Vincent Vinciguerra, MD, who heads the Don Monti Division of Hematology and Oncology at North Shore University Hospital, believes passionately in educating patients about how they can prevent cancer and eat healthfully while undergoing cancer treatment. "We offer a nutritional consultation free of charge," he says. That kind of service should be made available to all cancer patients through effective public policy, so that it becomes standard practice.

Beyond their role as advocates for their own patients, oncologists and other health care providers need to join broader efforts to infuse their field with a prevention orientation and confront the unsustainable costs of cancer care. The medical curriculum is a good place to start. Doctors in training should be steeped in the idea that medicine's overarching goal is to prevent disease from occurring, and the syllabus should be revised to place new emphasis on prevention and wellness care.

Professional societies should also be addressing the lack of optimal tests and techniques for the screening of most cancers, the scant oversight of off-label drug prescribing, and the promotion of exorbitantly priced cancer therapies that offer marginal benefits.

Organizations like the American Society of Clinical Oncology and the American Medical Association are powerful players in the health care system, and could be effective advocates for reform. They should be raising their voices in Washington on the topics of reimbursement, the misguided focus of current cancer research, and the importance of redirecting federal resources toward primary prevention and early detection.

Ultimately, we may need to make changes simply because we will run out of money if we continue our current approach to cancer.

One possible vehicle for navigating an alternative approach is the National Comprehensive Cancer Network (NCCN), a nonprofit alliance of 21 leading cancer centers that describes itself as "the arbiter of high-quality cancer care."[9] The network is in some ways more influential than the FDA in determining how drugs get used. Oncologists, cancer surgeons, and other cancer experts meet regularly in committees to review new research, current clinical practices, and novel therapies in order to develop practice guidelines. These guidelines help to establish a "standard of care" for doctors, which insurance companies then use to make decisions about covering screening tests, treatment, and other health services.

In its current mode, the NCCN is under no pressure to keep costs under control. Rather, its goal is to find "optimum" therapeutic pathways. The NCCN is not subject to federal oversight, and committee leaders differ in how flexible or rigid they are in issuing treatment guidelines. As a general rule, if there is evidence that a drug offers a clinical benefit, no matter how slight, it will likely win the NCCN's backing.

The medical community can advocate for a better approach. We would be much better served if the NCCN factored "value-based care" into its decision making and issued recommendations that benefited patients rather than the pharmaceutical industry. While we cannot fully replicate the United Kingdom's model of providing reimbursement only for drugs deemed cost-effective, the NCCN could acknowledge resource limitations in recommending standards of care.

If the medical community is unwilling to make those reforms, an initiative by the federal government to create a modified version of the UK's National Institute for Health and Clinical Excellence (NICE) may be the solution to this American dilemma. A "NICE-lite" initiative would be a way to use information about the cost and effectiveness of therapy to set standards for quality of care and to guide physicians' decision making. It could define "excellence" in a way that supports the needs of both patients and our entire society.

ADVOCATES SPEAK UP

The advocacy community is another critical player in promoting cancer prevention to the top of the nation's agenda. While the government has far greater resources for shaping the direction of cancer research, the on-the-ground knowledge and connections of advocates can help advance a broader effort. Many advocates first became involved after personal struggles of their own.

News anchor Katie Couric became a passionate advocate of colon cancer screening after her husband, Jay Monahan, succumbed to the disease at the age of 41. Couric decided to have her colonoscopy broadcast on television, and in what came to be known as the "Couric effect," the number of people who had a colonoscopy subsequently jumped by 20 percent.[10] Couric went on to establish the Entertainment Industry Foundation's National Colorectal Cancer Research Alliance, which has been highly effective in promoting colonoscopies and raising money for cutting-edge research.

Likewise, the strides against childhood leukemia since the 1970s demonstrate that advocacy matters. At that time, the deaths of two teenage boys, Don Monti and T.J. Martell, led their grieving parents to create research foundations to spare other families the agony of losing a child to cancer.

"Courage, grace and hope" are the guiding principles of the Don Monti Memorial Research Foundation. Caroline Monti Saladino, who lost her brother Don to leukemia, works tirelessly with her husband, Arthur, her brother Richard, and her children to fulfill the foundation's mission. "The health care facilities we support offer hope, compassion, and state-of-the-art treatment to cancer patients," she says. "We truly are making a difference." One of the groundbreaking studies this foundation supports, in partnership with the Cold Spring Harbor Laboratory, involves the use of genomic technologies to identify DNA changes that may contribute to leukemia.

The T.J. Martell Foundation is the music industry's largest foundation funding medical research for cancer and AIDS. It has drawn support from such musical luminaries as Ella Fitzgerald and Duke Ellington and has raised some $250 million to underwrite innovative cancer research across the country. "Ultimately, I'd like to dissolve the foundation because we've found a cure for cancer. Not to have a need for this foundation is my goal. That would be my way of striking back at cancer for taking my beloved son, T.J.," says Tony Martell, founder of the foundation and a former top executive at Epic Records.

The Lustgarten Foundation, the largest private foundation dedicated exclusively to funding pancreatic cancer research, reminds us how vital the corporate sector can be in raising resources. Established by Marc Lustgarten, the former vice chairman of Cablevision, who died of the disease at 52, as well as Cablevision chairman Charles Dolan and chief executive James Dolan, the Lustgarten Foundation has its administrative costs paid by Cablevision, allowing the foundation to devote 100 percent of its donations to research. Cablevision and the Lustgarten Foundation are also partners in a campaign, called curePC, to raise public awareness of pancreatic cancer.

Laurie C. Carson founded the Lung Cancer Research Foundation after losing both her brother, who had never smoked, and her uncle, who had quit 20 years before his death, to lung cancer. Better screening, ideally through a test that uses saliva or blood, and improved prevention and treatment are all foundation priorities. Carson sees cross-cutting partnerships as the way to reach those goals. When I asked her about the need for collaboration among cancer advocates, she responded without hesitation, "I believe that we could do more to support clinical efforts in partnership with universities and with the federal government. That hasn't happened so far."

That message of collaboration has been taken to heart within the breast cancer community, where numerous organizations have historically operated in separate silos. In 2007, the first-ever Collaborative Summit on Breast Cancer Research brought together representatives from 27 groups, and the summit has since become an annual event.[11] Collaboration is the only way forward, insists Ambassador Nancy G. Brinker, founder and CEO of Susan G. Komen for the Cure. "There are more organizations than there is revenue to supply everyone. We need to figure out how to work together better."

Just as we need team science, we also need "team advocacy" to use the resources, collective wisdom, creativity, and lobbying power of all the dedicated cancer activists we can bring together.

TAKING PERSONAL RESPONSIBILITY

Nothing about the importance of involving government, science, and advocates in the mission to create a cancer prevention agenda diminishes our responsibility as individuals. Each of us has a personal obligation to make the smartest decisions we can about our own health.

This is discussed more thoroughly in the next few chapters, but some basic guidelines are worth highlighting here.

Make the behavior changes proven to lower cancer risk. We begin with the obvious. Avoid tobacco; maintain a healthy body weight; eat more whole grains, vegetables, and fruits; and exercise. Reduce your intake of added sugar, which appears not only in soft drinks, snacks, and desserts but in many other processed foods as well. These are major steps toward reducing cancer risk, but too many of us fail to take them consistently.

In general, I am much more enthusiastic about whole foods and good nutrition than I am about taking supplements or about other therapies purported to prevent cancer. Vitamin D and calcium are the exceptions, where the science for supplementing your diet with a pill is strong.

Minimize your exposure to environmental contaminants and medical radiation. We don't yet know enough about the interaction of various chemicals or how much exposure over what period of time represents a real danger, but we do know that many products on the market contain known carcinogens. Buying organic foods, products packaged in BPA-free containers, cosmetics without parabens (widely used preservatives), and safer personal care and household cleaning products are good for your own health, and for the environment.

Discuss screening with your doctor. The colonoscopy is the gold standard for detecting colon cancer and its early warning signs, the Pap test has transformed the course of cervical cancer, and mammography remains the only tool we have to screen broad populations for breast cancer. Where the science is uncertain, become an informed consumer so that you and your doctor can make sound decisions about what screening tests are most suitable for your own health situation.

Take precautions in the sun. The sun's ultraviolet light can damage the cells, leading to genetic mutations that can cause skin cancer. Use sunscreen with a sun-protection factor (SPF) of at least 30, wear a brimmed hat and clothing that covers your arms and legs, and use wrap-around sunglasses that provide maximum protection. It is also important to seek shade, especially midday, when the sun's rays are strongest. Check your skin monthly for suspicious moles and lesions and take special care to protect your children, because sun damage early in life can show up decades later as skin cancer.

Get cancer-prevention vaccines. Ideally, all girls and boys should receive the three-dose human papillomavirus vaccine by age 11 or 12, according to the CDC. Since the vaccine has been on the market only since 2006, adolescents and young adults up to age 26 should also be vaccinated. The other cancer prophylactic is the hepatitis B vaccine, which helps to lower the risk of liver cancer.

Be part of the solution. Beyond actions designed to protect our health as individuals, there is much we can do as advocates. If your community still permits smoking in public places, does not provide safe opportunities to walk and play, or lacks options for purchasing fresh food, find out what nonprofit organizations are working on those issues in your area and sign up to help. If your school district allows the sale of soda and other sugar-rich foods lacking nutritional value in vending machines, get involved with the local PTA and insist that they be replaced with healthful alternatives.

If we can give young people the tools to lead healthier, more physically active lives, we can lower their cancer risk dramatically. Surely, we owe them no less. As the President's Cancer Panel declared in its 2008–2009 report: "To a greater extent than many realize, individuals have the power to affect public policy."[12]

CHAPTER 10

CANCER-PROOFING THE ENVIRONMENT

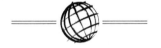

LMOST 80,000 CHEMICALS ARE SOLD IN THE United States, and we are exposed to many of them on a daily basis. We know with alarming certainty that some of these cause cancer, but most remain unexamined and largely unregulated.

"Research on environmental causes of cancer has been limited by low priority and inadequate funding," the President's Cancer Panel declared in its report released in April 2010, *Reducing Environmental Cancer Risk: What We Can Do Now.*[1] As a result, "the consequences of cumulative lifetime exposures to known carcinogens and the interaction of specific environmental contaminants remain largely unstudied."

From acetaldehyde and acid mists to wood dust and x-rays, the International Agency for Research on Cancer, part of the World Health Organization, states flatly that more than 100 agents in use today are "carcinogenic to humans." Several hundred others are classified as either "probably" or "possibly" carcinogenic to humans. The Environmental Protection Agency (EPA) and the National Toxicology Program also maintain separate and overlapping lists of cancer-causing substances.

Despite the obvious need for scientific expertise and appropriate regulation, staffing in the EPA offices most responsible for overseeing toxic substances has dropped considerably in recent years. The cutbacks are probably due to some combination of ideological resistance to government intervention and resource shortfalls. Two years after the President's Cancer Panel issued powerful and specific recommendations for reducing the cancer risks in the environment, I see little to indicate that we have started to implement them.

DANGERS OF SPECIAL CONCERN

Contaminants in the environment can disrupt the normal functioning of the body's genetic, immune, and endocrine systems and promote the mutations in a cell's DNA that result in cancer. While all of that is established scientific fact, we know much less about the mix of environmental hazards that truly put us at risk. Part of the difficulty in establishing danger has been a tendency to focus on acute, high doses of single agents, when it may be the cumulative effects of long-term, low-level, or combination exposures that put us at greatest risk.

Tragically, chemical exposures may well be partially responsible for the rise in invasive cancers among young people. The growth in childhood cancers has been slow but steady, averaging about 0.5 percent annually since 1975, according to the American Cancer Society (ACS).[2] Yet, we haven't devoted the necessary resources to understand exactly why this is happening.

We do know that the developing bodies of children make them more susceptible to environmental carcinogens and compounds. Along with having a greater sensitivity to initial exposure, infants and children are less able to repair the damage contaminants can cause to various systems of the body, including the nervous, immune, respiratory, and reproductive systems.[3] Indeed, the President's Cancer Panel said that given the ability of environmental contaminants to cross the placental barrier to reach the fetus, babies are, in essence, being "pre-polluted."

Many experts think the consequences are clear. At least some childhood cancers "can be traced back to damage done at the cellular level from chemicals that are carcinogens," asserts Richard Clapp, DSc, MPH, professor emeritus of environmental science at Boston University School of Public Health. "There are a number of chemical exposures for which the evidence is strong, including leukemia and brain cancer."[4] Those two types account for more than half of all childhood cancers.

Neither the National Cancer Institute (NCI) nor the ACS has raised special alarm about the higher incidence of childhood cancer. Instead, they emphasize the triumphs of treatment. It is true that we have made real strides here, with mortality rates declining by two-thirds over the past 40 years. Nonetheless, cancer remains the second leading cause of death in children, after accidents, and the failure to find out why is appalling.

The sluggish pace at which government is responding to three environmental dangers—bisphenol A (BPA), perchloroethylene (perc), and parabens—has generated particular concern. Among many other chemicals in wide household use, these may or may not actually pose the gravest danger to human health, and that's part of the problem—we just don't know.

BPA is ubiquitous in consumer products, including plastic bottles and the inside coating of cans containing food. A growing body of research suggests there may be links between BPA and cancer. A recent study published in *Environmental Health Perspective,* for example, found that low levels of BPA had the capacity to activate pathways associated with the growth of cancer in mice.[5] On its Web site, the Environmental Working Group, a nonprofit organization dedicated to protecting public health and the environment, describes a number of other studies that show BPA's adverse health effects in animals.[6]

Although the European Union has banned BPA in baby bottles, there are no restrictions on its use in the United States. An eagerly awaited FDA assessment of BPA surprised many experts when it was released in March 2012. The agency downplayed the possible risk, although it promised to continue studying the chemical. Meanwhile, it showed a remarkable deference to industry as it described the steps being taken to reduce human exposure to BPA in the food supply. These steps, the agency wrote, include "supporting the industry's actions to stop producing BPA-containing baby bottles and infant feeding cups for the U.S. market" and "supporting efforts to replace BPA or minimize BPA levels in other food can linings."

If the agency believes BPA poses enough danger to support

industry's voluntary efforts, then the FDA should insist that industry act. That's what it means to be a good steward of the public's health.

Another example of the government taking limited steps when more aggressive action is called for is the EPA's approach to perchloroethylene, the chemical solvent widely used in dry cleaning. The agency has called perc a "likely human carcinogen."[7] Animal studies show that it causes cancer in rats that inhale or ingest it, and dry-cleaning industry workers have an elevated risk of certain cancers (including bladder cancer, non-Hodgkin's lymphoma, and multiple myeloma). Recognizing the risk to people who live or work in a building where a dry cleaner is housed, the EPA has issued rules banning perc's use in residential buildings. However, those rules don't go into effect until 2020, an unjustified delay given that the agency acknowledges the danger.

The Natural Resources Defense Council, an environmental action group based in New York City, thinks the evidence is strong enough to recommend that consumers use other methods to clean their clothes. Nontoxic, noncarcinogenic options are available, which means the EPA could begin phasing out perc in commercial cleaning altogether.

Parabens are a third area of concern. These preservatives are used in a wide variety of cosmetics, moisturizers, hair care products, and shaving items, but are no longer present in most deodorants. They can also be found in food, including processed meats, certain snacks and candy, and some liquid dietary supplements, as well as in some prescription drugs. Where manufacturers are required to list ingredients on the label, as they are with cosmetics and food, these products may appear as methylparaben, propylparaben, butylparaben, or benzylparaben, among others.

Parabens have weak estrogen-like properties, suggesting the possibility that they could stimulate the growth of hormone-related cancers. A number of studies have found traces of parabens in breast tumors, although a cause-and-effect relationship has not been established.[8] FDA officials have told consumers they need not be concerned, while offering the agency's pro forma promise to evaluate new research as it becomes available.[9] A more engaged strategy would be to urge the appropriate federal scientific agencies to conduct the research themselves. What are we waiting for?

Then there is medical radiation, which can increase the risk of cancer. Many people don't realize how much exposure they get from the imaging technology that has transformed medical care.

The radiation dose from a CT scan is equivalent to the dose resulting from between 100 and 800 chest x-rays, depending on where in the body it is performed and why.[10] In the early 1980s, about 3.3 million CT scans were being performed every year. By 2010 that number had risen to 80 million.[11] This represents a 24-fold increase in medical radiation exposure to the US population. Other tests supply radiation at even higher levels—positron emission tomography (PET) can have a radiation dose equivalent to as many as 2,000 chest x-rays.[12]

Used appropriately, all this equipment has essential medical value for screening and diagnostic purposes because it allows us to visualize parts of the body in three-dimensional detail. However, physicians are generally on their own to prescribe imaging tests as they see fit, and some of the factors that can influence their decisions—including concerns about litigation and having an ownership stake in the costly equipment—may not address the best interests of the patient. "CT scans account for a large proportion of medical radiation exposure to people over a lifetime," says Dr. Barnett Kramer, director of the NCI's Division of Prevention. "In many cases, they are done without clear proof of benefit."

The medical community should create consistent guidelines to help physicians decide whether an imaging test is appropriate. Also, poor record keeping means physicians may not be able to access a patient's medical history across clinical settings. If they don't know what tests a patient has already had and how much radiation he or she has received in the past, they may order repeat tests that could have been avoided.

While the radiation risk from imaging technology to any given individual is small, the cumulative impact is not—the 70 million CT scans performed in 2007 can be expected to cause some 15,000 to 45,000 new cancers, according to a calculation in *Archives of Internal Medicine*.[13] The Institute of Medicine (IOM) says there is "consistent evidence" for a link between breast cancer and ionizing radiation.[14]

Along with overuse, the medical imaging system is plagued by problems of inconsistent dosing. The lack of standardization was dramatized in a study showing an average 13-fold variation between the highest and lowest doses of radiation administered for the same test. That certainly suggests some doctors are using more radiation than necessary to get the information they need.[15]

In 2010, the FDA launched the Initiative to Reduce Unnecessary Radiation Exposure from Medical Imaging to address some of these issues.[16] The American public and advocacy groups should be closely monitoring its activities to ensure that it does what is necessary to limit the cancer risks of medical radiation.

BPA, perc, parabens, and medical radiation are among the most discussed environmental risk factors associated with cancer, but they aren't the only ones.

The IOM has identified benzene, ethylene oxide, and 1,3-butadiene as chemicals that may be associated with breast cancer.[17] Other cancer-causing contaminants in industrial settings have seeped into the soil, air, and water to which entire populations are exposed. Likewise, carcinogenic agricultural fertilizers and pesticides have entered the water supply in many locations. We are also exposed to toxins on a daily basis through particulates in the air, motor vehicle exhaust, cleaning chemicals, and disinfectants intended to improve drinking-water safety.

In all likelihood "the true burden of environmentally induced cancer has been grossly underestimated," according to the President's Cancer Panel report. One barrier to more studies is the fragmentation across agencies charged with protecting the environment, including the EPA, the FDA, the Consumer Product Safety Commission, and other federal agencies, which mirrors the fragmentation across the cancer establishment. The panel said that "a more integrated, coordinated and transparent system . . . driven by science and free of political or industry influence" is needed to develop and enforce regulations.

As the system stands, we lack uniform standards for measuring and classifying contaminants across government agencies, and there is no agreement on the levels of exposure that justify concern. We know far too little about the low-dose chronic exposures to chemical combinations that may affect the largest populations. Good studies are also challenged by the long latency period that exists between exposures and most cancers, which makes it difficult to tease out cause and effect.

For the most part, we now regulate chemicals by allowing them to be used, and then reacting if evidence of a problem accumulates. Requiring manufacturers to prove their products safe before marketing them would be a huge step forward in making a prevention-oriented commitment.

As a physician, I would also like to see my own community of medical professionals step forward more boldly on the issue of environmental toxins and demand that the federal government fund additional research and regulate contaminants that pose risks. Doctors should also remember to consider occupational and environmental exposures when diagnosing illness, and do more to make their patients aware of how they can protect themselves. Our professional societies should be taking the lead to accomplish this goal.

The Need for Government Action

The President's Cancer Panel offered numerous ideas for pushing an adequately funded research agenda forward and for limiting our exposure to toxins. Here are some of this compelling report's most important conclusions and recommendations:

We need to learn more. We should be improving our measurement tools and collecting better data on exposure, deepening our understanding of the interactions among contaminants, and studying the magnitude of the cancer risk much more rigorously. Right now, we lack the science to understand what lifelong exposures to various combinations of chemicals do to us.

Environmental health should be integrated into the nation's disease prevention agenda. When we make policy decisions—for example, about how to fund health services, how to improve access to care, or what public health measures to introduce—environmental exposures and their impact on disease should be carefully considered. This reform is long overdue.

We owe our children more protection. We know that children are at special risk from environmental contaminants, but we don't have an adequate understanding of the threats. Nor do we have an adequate number of researchers and clinicians trained in pediatric environmental health. What we do know is that our failure to act against cancer-promoting contamination is having a profound effect on children.

We must act with a sense of urgency. Animal and laboratory studies can tell us a lot about human risk. The long delays between environmental exposure and the development of cancer obligate us to develop a framework for protecting people on the basis of what we learn in the lab. If we wait for cause-and-effect relationships to be established in humans before we act, we are waiting too long.

Our approach to environmental regulations needs to be updated. The current system for assessing and regulating contaminants is overly complex, weak, and fragmented. As a result, many known or suspected carcinogens are escaping the nation's watchdogs altogether.

We can reduce exposure to medical radiation. With stricter regulations and more professional guidelines, we can instruct physicians to use imaging technology less often and to use lower doses of radiation to get the same diagnostic information.

We don't talk enough about cancer-promoting exposures in the workplace. Too often, we have not been honest with agricultural and industrial workers about their occupational risks. Nor do we always alert communities when these exposures contaminate their air, water, or soil. Without disclosure, people cannot protect themselves when possible or seek timely medical care when necessary.

Alternatives to carcinogenic chemicals are available. Many products can be reformulated to use safer ingredients, but government needs to create carrot-and-stick incentives to get industry to do so.

Protecting Yourself

While we advocate for more aggressive action from government, we also need to take more initiative ourselves to mitigate the risks of carcinogens in the environment. Even if the science is inconclusive and the regulators aren't ready to act, there are plenty of precautions we can take. Here are some guidelines.

Reduce contaminants at home. Make choices about food, cleaning products, toys, and medicine that minimize household exposure. Eat organic foods and avoid additives, clean with products that use organic ingredients instead of chemicals, filter tap water, and ban smoking in the home. Check the ingredients on your personal grooming products for parabens, which should be avoided. Use organic herbicides or fertilizer on your lawn. Remove your shoes and wash work clothes separately from household laundry to keep workplace contaminants out of the home.

Avoid BPA. Because BPA can leach into food from plastic

containers and cans, it is best to avoid those as much as possible. Look for cans labeled BPA-free and plastic containers with recycling labels #1, #2, and #4, which do not contain the chemical. Avoid the #7 label, which often does. Use stainless steel and glass containers for storing food, and don't microwave food in plastics containing BPA.

Minimize dry cleaning. The National Resources Defense Council suggests seeking out cleaners that use alternate methods, including wet cleaning or liquid carbon dioxide. If you do use a conventional dry cleaner, remove the plastic bag that covers your clothes and air them out for several hours before hanging them in your closet or putting them on your body.

Make informed decisions about medical radiation. Ask your doctor why an imaging test is recommended and whether it is really necessary. "You need to know how the CT scan will improve your outcomes," advises Dr. Kramer. "You also want to keep track of how many scans and x-rays you've had." It is reasonable to ask whether an alternative test that does not use radiation, such as an MRI or a sonagram, can provide the necessary information.

Keep your own records of any imaging tests you have. Indicate the date of the test and who performed it, so that other doctors need not repeat the same tests.

Limit cell phone use. Cell phones use radiofrequency waves, a form of electromagnetism that has been classified as "possibly carcinogenic to humans" by the International Agency for Research on Cancer. A link between cell phone use and brain tumors has not been established, but the US National Toxicology Program is conducting its largest research study ever to find out whether cell phones have toxic or carcinogenic effects.

Meanwhile, it makes sense to take precautions. The general rule is to keep your phone distant from your brain, either with a headset, speakerphone, or Bluetooth device, or by texting instead of calling. Limit children's use of cell phones. You can also look for a phone with a lower specific absorption rate (SAR), which is a measure of the level of radiofrequency energy it emits. Comparative SAR charts are available on the Internet, including on the CNET Web site (www.cnet.com).

Become an advocate. Americans need to speak out about the importance of studying environmental contaminants and their links to cancer and about regulating those that are dangerous. Let your elected representatives know that you expect government to fulfill its obligation to public health. When you make the choice to purchase nontoxic consumer products, contact the manufacturers and let them know that you are supporting safer products.

———

With its clarion call for high-level leadership to reduce environmental contaminants, the President's Cancer Panel reminded us that Americans have the right to expect adequate protection from their government. Addressing the president directly, the Panel wrote: "The grievous harm from this group of carcinogens has not been addressed adequately. . . . The American people—even before they are born—are bombarded continually with myriad combinations of these dangerous exposures.

"The Panel urges you most strongly to use the power of your office to remove the carcinogens and other toxins from our food, water, and air that needlessly increase health care costs, cripple our Nation's productivity, and devastate American lives."

CHAPTER 11

ENDING THE SCOURGE OF TOBACCO

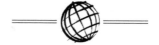

THE DANGERS OF TOBACCO HAVE BEEN THE subject of aggressive public health action at every level of government. These efforts have led to a well-documented decline in the adult smoking rate and have encouraged fewer young people to take up the habit. Nonetheless, smoking remains the leading source of preventable death in the United States and the cause of one-third of all cancers.[1] Further reductions in tobacco use will require an escalated commitment by local, state, and federal governments and by the private sector.

While the relationship between smoking and lung cancer is well known, smoking's association with other cancers is not so widely recognized. A 2004 Surgeon General's report linked smoking to cancers of the bladder, cervix, esophagus, kidney, larynx, throat, mouth, nasal cavity, pancreas, and stomach, as well as to acute myeloid leukemia.[2] All that, of course, is in addition to the other damage that tobacco does to the lungs, heart, and other organs.

A connection to colorectal cancer has been documented more recently. Research published in the *American Journal of Epidemiology* in 2009 found that women who had smoked the equivalent of 10 "pack years" before age 30 increased their risk of colon cancer by 16 percent, compared with nonsmokers.[3] (A pack year is the number of years a person has smoked an average of one pack of cigarettes per day.)

Secondhand smoke also does terrible harm. "Sufficient evidence" exists to tie secondhand smoke to lung cancer in adults, and there is "suggestive evidence" of a link to breast, nasal, and sinus-related cancers, according to *The Tobacco Atlas*, a compendium jointly published by the American Cancer Society and the World Lung Foundation. "Suggestive evidence" indicates that children exposed to secondhand smoke have an increased chance of developing brain tumors, lymphoma, and leukemia.

None of that damage should surprise us, given that tobacco smoke contains some 7,000 chemicals, at least 69 of which are known to cause cancer. Among these are arsenic and DDT, which are also found in some insecticides; toluene, an industrial solvent; acetylene, used in welding torches; and formaldehyde.[4]

Despite decades of warnings, almost 20 percent of the adult population—45.3 million people age 18 or older—still smokes.[5] This is a considerable decline from the early 1970s, when at least

40 percent of adults were smokers, but it's not nearly enough.[6] The need to stop young people from taking up the habit is especially urgent. Every day in the United States, almost 4,000 people under age 18 smoke their first cigarette, and about 1,000 of them will become daily smokers. Many are also partial to cigars and smokeless tobacco.[7]

Less educated people are most likely to smoke, making the associated health risks still another penalty of being disadvantaged. Forty-five percent of adults with a GED diploma smoke, as do one-third of adults with less than a high-school education—compared with just 6 percent of adults who have a graduate degree and 10 percent of adults with a college diploma. We see the same general pattern through the lens of income: Almost 29 percent of adults living below the poverty line are smokers, compared with 18 percent of higher-income adults.[8]

Nicotine is the addictive ingredient in tobacco, and the reason people keep on smoking against all common sense, or fail to quit despite a desperate desire to do so. The FDA has called cigarettes "nicotine-delivery devices," and numerous internal documents attest to industry's elaborate efforts to breed more nicotine into tobacco.[9]

Indeed, it is such a powerful drug that some smokers continue the habit even after they have been diagnosed with lung cancer—14 to 18 percent do so, according to one study. Perhaps they conclude that they will gain little by stopping once they are ill, but they are wrong—quitting even at the time of diagnosis significantly enhances the chances of survival.[10]

"Persistent smoking will affect the cancer patient's treatment outcome," says Carolyn Dresler, MD, MPA, who chairs the Tobacco Control Subcommittee of the American Society of Clinical Oncologists. She is frustrated that even physicians don't always recognize this. When a well-known oncologist told her, "It's too late—they already have cancer," Dr. Dresler was aghast. "What do you mean, it's too late?" she responded. "The patient's response to therapy will be affected by the smoking. It's never too late!"

Beyond the terrible toll in cancer and other health problems, smoking is enormously costly to society. Annual public and private health care costs alone are about $96 billion, and lost productivity resulting from lives cut short by smoking-related deaths adds $97 billion more to the total, according to the Campaign for Tobacco-Free Kids, one of the nation's foremost tobacco control organizations.[11]

———

Against this bleak news, one hopeful fact stands out: Tobacco is an enemy that can be defeated—a "winnable battle," as the Centers for Disease Control and Prevention (CDC) has called it. Numerous tobacco-control measures have been carefully evaluated, and we have the research to tell us what works. Aggressive health education campaigns, excise tax increases, increasingly stringent restrictions against smoking in public places, and shifts in social norms that make smoking unacceptable in many circles all help explain the significant decline in tobacco use that we have seen over the past few decades. These kinds of interventions also offer us models to use in our continuing efforts to influence other health behaviors linked to cancer.

Further progress in the tobacco arena demands commitment and funding, along with the recognition that the tobacco industry is still formidable and insidious. The climate has grown more hostile to its products, but none of us should be lulled into thinking that the tobacco companies will quietly concede defeat.

Tobacco control advocates will likely continue to face an adversary that is remarkably adept at developing highly addictive new products.

ADVOCATES TAKE ON THE INDUSTRY

Efforts to curb the tobacco industry's influence have been almost a century in the making. Hints of the health harms of smoking began to accumulate in the 1930s, although definitive evidence became widely available only when the Surgeon General released the *Report on Smoking and Health* in 1964.[12] The report confirmed the link between smoking and lung cancer, as well as a host of other diseases, and tobacco control began to gather momentum. Within a year, the first warning labels were required on cigarette packs, and by 1971 cigarette ads were no longer permitted on television.

The 1986 Surgeon General's report documenting the dangers of secondhand smoke—also called "forced smoking"—further ramped up concerns with its assertion that "there is no risk-free level of exposure to secondhand smoke."[13] Gradually, smoking has been banned in public spaces such as airplanes, most public transit systems, and office buildings, as well as restaurants and bars in many states.

In 1998, four leading cigarette manufacturers signed the Master Settlement Agreement (MSA) with the attorneys general of 46 states. The agreement, the largest civil litigation settlement in US history, released the companies from an onslaught of liability claims in exchange for payments to the states of some $200 billion over 25 years. In addition, the agreement placed new restrictions on marketing and advertising, compelled the industry to release many of its internal documents, and contributed $300 million a year for five years to fund the American Legacy Foundation to reduce youth smoking and provide public education. Subsequently, some 40 smaller cigarette companies signed on to the MSA, meaning virtually the entire domestic tobacco industry now complies with its terms.[14]

While the MSA was a major step toward forcing the industry to acknowledge the harm it had done, it also had limitations. The agreement contained no explicit provisions requiring the states to use any portion of the settlement funds specifically for tobacco control, and in an era of tight budgets, most of the revenues have been siphoned off for other government functions.

According to the CDC, states collected $25.3 billion in a combination of legal settlement funds and tobacco taxes in 2011, but spent less than 2 percent of that amount on efforts to curb tobacco use. Increasing the funds dedicated to prevention and control to a modest 15 percent would generate $3.7 billion, which is what the CDC says is necessary to fund state tobacco-control programs at recommended levels.[15] If we don't dedicate adequate resources to combat tobacco's lure for our youths and adults, more victims will succumb to lung and other cancers.

A promising development is the Family Prevention and Tobacco Control Act, passed by Congress in 2009, which gives the FDA the authority to regulate the manufacture and sale of tobacco products. As a result, we will be seeing a new generation of larger and more explicit graphic warning labels on cigarettes; more aggressive efforts to curb tobacco marketing and sales to children; bans on deceptive product claims, such as "light" and "low-tar"; and prohibitions against candy- and fruit-flavored cigarettes designed specifically to appeal to children.

The shifting regulatory landscape is clearly making it more difficult and more expensive for the tobacco companies to sell their products, and yet, the industry will not readily give up its stranglehold on Americans. It has a long track record of finding new opportunities to sell its products when old channels are closed off. Despite increasingly restrictive limits on advertising and promotion, the companies spent almost $10 billion in 2008 to market cigarettes in the United States alone.[16] A disproportionate amount of this money was spent on advertising that targets African American and low-income youths.[17]

The industry retains that kind of clout at least partly because it lobbies extensively and contributes generously to the political campaigns of both parties. *The Tobacco Atlas* reports that in 2010 the Altria Group/Philip Morris spent more than $10 million on lobbying in the United States. Tobacco companies contributed $3.1 million to federal election campaigns that year—$2.1 million to Republicans and $1 million to Democrats.[18] Just how such donations influence public policy is difficult to assess, but it is safe to assume the industry thinks it is getting something for its money.

RENEWING A COMMITMENT TO TOBACCO CONTROL

The unfinished business of tobacco control will advance dramatically if an ambitious interagency federal plan, Ending the Tobacco Epidemic: A Tobacco Control Strategic Action Plan, released in 2010, is actually translated into action. The Campaign for Tobacco-Free Kids calls it the "first truly comprehensive initiative to reduce tobacco use since the 1964 Surgeon General's report."[19]

Guided by the Department of Health and Human Services, the plan lays out a series of "high-impact interventions that include smoke-free air for everyone, tobacco price increases, an adequately funded mass-media educational campaign, and full access to comprehensive tobacco cessation services." The federal government proposes to increase financial support and technical assistance to the states so they can expand their quit-smoking programs, implement policies that further restrict youths' access to tobacco, and promote the benefits of smoke-free laws. Strategies for changing social norms around tobacco are also part of the plan, which calls for hard-hitting educational campaigns targeted at multiple audiences, and outreach to encourage leaders in the sports and entertainment industries to take a stand against smoking.

In addition, there are proposed measures to expand Medicaid and Medicare coverage for comprehensive cessation treatment and to provide incentives so that health care providers do a better job of educating their patients about tobacco and providing support for those who want to quit. To ensure that its interventions are timely and relevant, the plan also calls for a monitoring of evolving industry practices, public perceptions, and changes in tobacco products. Ongoing research is also emphasized to ensure that all action is grounded in scientific evidence. Learning more about which interventions work best with vulnerable and high-risk populations is a particular research priority.

The plan's stated intent is to "reinvigorate national momentum toward tobacco prevention and control by applying proven methods for reducing the burden of tobacco dependence." Actions are, of course, "subject to the availability of resources," as the plan itself acknowledges.

Let's make that investment. Taken together, the actions in the plan could reduce the rate of adult smoking to 12 percent by 2020.

———

Excise taxes are one of the most effective tobacco control strategies available. This is especially true in curbing adolescent smoking, because young people are so sensitive to costs. "You need to raise the price of tobacco," emphasizes Dr. Dresler. "Raise it a lot—make the price high so that kids can't buy the cigarettes. Youth respond well to higher taxes on cigarettes, because they can't afford the high prices."

Every 10 percent increase in the price of cigarettes reduces overall consumption by about 3 to 5 percent. The tobacco companies themselves know that taxes will affect their sales, and they are afraid of that. "Of all the concerns, there is one—taxation—that alarms us the most," acknowledged Altria/Philip Morris in one of its internal documents.[20]

In 2009, the federal tobacco tax was increased by 62 cents, bringing the total tax to $1.01, and that same year, cigarette sales dropped by more than 8 percent. State taxes, which average $1.45 per pack, add considerably more to the price, although these vary by state. New York has the highest state tax in the nation, at $4.35 per pack, while Missouri has the lowest, at just 17 cents. In general, taxes on other tobacco products, including smokeless tobacco, tend to be much lower.

In the first decade of the 21st century, an average of 10 states a year increased their cigarette taxes, but this trend has slowed in the past few years, with just 3 states enacting small increases in 2011. New Hampshire actually lowered its tax by 10 cents.[21]

Matthew Myers, president of the Campaign for Tobacco-Free Kids, warns that "the failure to increase cigarette taxes is part of a broader backsliding in the states' efforts to reduce tobacco use." States cut $260 million from their prevention and cessation budgets from 2008 through 2011, spending less on tobacco prevention in 2011 than at any time since they first began receiving funds from the tobacco settlement.[22] Coincident with those cuts, the progress made in reducing tobacco use among high school students began to slow.[23]

Restricting smoking in public places is another core tobacco control strategy because it works on two levels, protecting non-smokers from tobacco exposure while also encouraging smokers to quit. The Campaign for Tobacco-Free Kids reviewed the body of research on this topic and concluded that workplace restrictions lead smokers to smoke less, to make more attempts to quit, and ultimately to be more likely to quit. The organization also found that young people were less likely to smoke if they lived in communities that banned all smoking in restaurants and that smoke-free housing on college campuses discouraged nonsmokers from taking up the habit.[24]

At present, 29 states, hundreds of municipalities, and Washington, DC, Puerto Rico, and the US Virgin Islands have smoke-free laws that keep tobacco out of most bars and restaurants.[25] The tobacco industry lobbied aggressively against most of these laws, working systematically, state by state and city by city, as legislation was introduced and debated. Its claims about the harm such laws would do to businesses were misleading, given the many studies consistently showing that such laws "do not adversely affect business revenue or operating costs." Indeed, some surveys suggest people eat out *more* often where smoking is not permitted.[26] With that kind of evidence, the remaining states should act now to end smoking where food and drink are served.

Graphic warnings are another powerful tobacco-control strategy, and an important component of the FDA's regulatory approach under the Tobacco Control Act. Beginning in September 2012, cigarette packs are to carry nine explicit textual warnings on a rotating basis, including such messages as "Smoking can kill you" and "Cigarettes cause cancer." In addition, color graphics illustrating the harms of smoking will be required to cover the top half of the front and rear panels of the package. The images are dramatic—a man with rotting teeth, a baby breathing in her mother's smoke, healthy pink lungs contrasted with mottled, disfigured ones. Any ad for cigarettes appearing in media or poster formats will be required to carry a warning that covers at least 20 percent of the ad.[27]

Predictably, the tobacco companies have filed suit, claiming that these requirements violate their rights of free speech. Although a lower court sided with the industry, the US Court of Appeals for the Sixth Circuit ruled in March 2012 that the requirement to use the graphic warnings was legal. Hopefully, that ruling is upheld if the industry decides to continue fighting through the judicial system.

Beyond the realm of the public sector, there are many opportunities to engage the medical and scientific communities, schools, private employers, and others in stamping out tobacco use.

Doctors can play an important role in encouraging their patients not to smoke, but many avoid the topic altogether. Dr. Dresler told me several disturbing stories about physicians who did not counsel their patients appropriately against tobacco use.

One physician said that he avoided such conversations because he wouldn't be reimbursed for his time. Another feared that his patients wouldn't return for care if he spoke too harshly against tobacco. "If I push for smoking cessation, they'll get angry, and they won't come back and see me," this doctor commented. A prominent breast oncologist who said he did not talk about tobacco use with his patients had a truly astounding rationale for avoiding the discussion: He felt that his breast cancer patients were already too stressed out by their diagnosis and treatment and did not need something else to worry about.

Those kinds of responses are simply unacceptable. As Dr. Dresler observes, we would never permit such excuses to delay action in the face of other threats. "If a person has a blood glucose level of 400, would they not address it? If a person has blood pressure over 120, would they not address it?" Obviously, most doctors would act in those circumstances, yet too many have somehow justified a different standard when it comes to tobacco. "If you have a patient in front of you with a deadly form of behavior addiction, then it is unethical not to address it," she insists.

Doctors who encourage their patients not to smoke can have a meaningful impact, which makes their avoidance of appropriate interventions all the more puzzling. Indeed, Dr. Dresler encourages doctors to use the US Tobacco Use Guidelines, a well-documented intervention known as the "5 A's"—ask, advise, assess, assist, and arrange—which, evidence tells us, helps people to stop smoking. By talking to patients about their smoking habits, impressing on them the value of quitting, and guiding them to treatments that help them do so, doctors remain true to their calling, which is to save lives.

Educational institutions are another venue where we can do more. Although some schools are already teaching the dangers of cigarette smoking in age-appropriate ways, all should do so at every grade level. The message should continue in college, when most students are of the legal age to buy cigarettes. Also on campus, college radio and television stations, printed material, and Web sites should all be used to promote cessation and refer students to programs that will help them quit.

Influential public figures admired by children, including well-known adolescent actors, should be speaking out bluntly against tobacco use in public service announcements and other forums. Vivid images of patients of all ages with asthma and various cancers would be very effective in making the point that tobacco is deadly.

The entertainment industry should pledge to remove images of people smoking from television programs, movies, music videos, video games, and other visual media.

Health insurance companies should routinely cover the costs of smoking cessation programs and treatment, and employers should offer incentives to employees who quit. I'd also like to see the NCI and other research funders take the lead in requiring scientists not to accept money from tobacco companies or their subsidiaries as a condition of their grants. Likewise, candidates for political office should refuse to accept campaign contributions from the tobacco industry and talk publicly about why.

Sadly, we're not likely to see the day when the use of tobacco is completely eliminated, along with the many cancers and other diseases it causes. However, by reinforcing our existing antismoking efforts and continuing to implement new ones, we can make great strides in the quest to be free of the scourge of tobacco.

CHAPTER 12

FIGHTING CANCER WITH NUTRITION AND PHYSICAL ACTIVITY

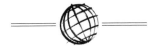

TOGETHER, OBESITY, DIET, AND LACK OF EXER-cise account for 30 percent of cancer in the United States. Obesity alone is responsible for one in every five cancers.[1] "We know that obesity causes breast and colon cancer," states Dr. Larry Norton of Memorial Sloan-Kettering Cancer Center.

Numerous studies document his assertion and highlight other links as well. A study published in the *New England Journal of Medicine*, for example, reported higher death rates from at least

14 different kinds of cancer among overweight populations. Over-all, the heaviest people were more than 50 percent more likely to die from cancer than normal-weight individuals.[2]

In a nation where more than one in three American adults is obese, we are clearly missing an opportunity to prevent cancer. Worse, we are imposing risks on future generations. There are 12.5 million obese children in the United States—about 17 percent of the population between the ages of 2 and 19.[3]

Obesity can increase the risk of cancer in many ways, according to the National Cancer Institute. We know, for example, that fat tissue produces excess estrogen, which is linked to the development of breast cancer. Fat cells also produce hormones that interact to regulate our metabolism. Leptin has been shown to have a pro-inflammatory effect, while adiponectin is anti-inflammatory. The link between inflammation and cancer is under investigation.

To keep cancer at bay, we need to work harder to end the nation's obesity epidemic. The solutions we most often hear about are encouraging individuals to take greater responsibility and motivating physicians to educate their patients about why good diet and exercise habits matter. While those steps are important, the truth is that much more has to be done to help people change the way they live.

As good stewards of public health, our local, state, and federal governments should help make nutritious foods and opportunities to exercise more widely available. Right now, residents of many communities don't feel safe walking in their neighborhoods, and many cash-strapped municipalities aren't providing safe places for children to play. Food deserts—neighborhoods or even entire towns where it is almost impossible to find fruits, vegetables, and other healthy foods so essential to cancer prevention—dot the landscape in urban and rural areas. Too many schools still allow children to purchase soda and candy from vending machines and have been canceling sports and other recreational activities because of tight budgets.

Many of our social norms add to the challenge of healthy living. It is common practice for workplace meetings to begin with a platter of high-fat muffins and white-flour doughnuts. The temptations of fat, sugar, and salt greet us everywhere—in restaurants, grocery stores, and coffee shops along with gas stations, pharmacies, and the pantries of our own homes.

Changing the status quo requires a new mind-set and new norms of what is good and acceptable at home, work, and play. Let's get started.

PUBLIC POLICIES TO PROMOTE HEALTHY LIVING

The basic guideline for physical activity is clear: Get moving. Exercise may be the most effective, least costly anticancer strategy we have. The Centers for Disease Control and Prevention (CDC) tells us that adults should get at least 2½ hours of moderate-intensity aerobic activity every week, plus muscle-strengthening activities at least twice a week. Children need more—at least an hour of physical activity daily.

The cancer-prevention impact is powerful. A look at almost 65,000 participants in the Harvard Nurses' Health Study found that premenopausal women who are very physically active—defined as running 3¼ hours per week or walking 13 hours per week—reduced their risk of breast cancer by 23 percent.[4] A study published in *Medicine and Science in Sports and Exercise* reported that 30 to

60 minutes of daily exercise reduced the risk of colon cancer by 30 to 40 percent and breast cancer by 20 to 30 percent.[5]

Yet more than one-quarter of US adults are not physically active during their leisure time, and only 2 in 10 get the CDC-recommended amounts of exercise.[6] If everyone could join a gym, that would be great, but we also need to consider how we can design communities that make it easier to be physically active.

Toward that goal, there is attention being paid to how we approach the built environment—the streets, residences, workplaces, schools, shops, and recreational facilities of our communities. Intelligent zoning regulations, urban planning decisions, and good transportation can all help us incorporate exercise into our daily lives.

The American Academy of Pediatrics has endorsed a package of recommendations that calls on pediatricians to advocate for these kinds of improvements and also asks local, state, and federal governments to do more to promote and fund active living.[7] Opportunities include building sidewalks, creating walking trails, encouraging mixed land use and higher-density neighborhoods that reduce sprawl, and locating schools and public buildings in easy-to-reach locations. Safe, well-lit parks can draw in local residents with activities throughout the day and evening.

We are also seeing some state legislation designed to put more exercise into our daily lives.[8] Some states have provided funds for bike and pedestrian pathways, required mass transit systems to allow bikes, and granted tax deductions to commuters who use public transportation or who bike to work. In many locales, there are laws establishing standards for physical education at all grade levels and protecting recess as a required part of the school day. Some legislation also places more attention on "complete streets," which factor in the needs of pedestrians, children, seniors, disabled populations, bicyclists, and mass transit users, as well as those of drivers, in roadway design.

These kinds of tangible, physical activity–promoting steps put prevention first, and are likely to have an impact on cancer risks. We need to expand all of them.

There has also been a limited but meaningful commitment of public resources to improve the quality of our food—a welcome foundation on which to build.

Many states now mandate nutrition education in schools. Exposing children to sound nutritional principles and teaching them to read food labels empowers them to make healthier choices. California has banned deep-fried foods from school cafeterias, Michigan encourages schools to purchase produce from local farms, and Rhode Island allows only healthy beverages and snacks to be sold in school vending machines.

In New York, the FreshConnect program, created in 2011, expanded farmers' markets to communities lacking access to fresh, local food. These markets also accept food stamps and other forms of nutritional assistance available to poor families and senior citizens, offering new food options to disadvantaged populations.[9]

Innovative strategies such as these can help transform lives.

On the federal level, other activities are under way to bring healthy food to communities without enough of it. A $400 million federal Healthy Food Financing Initiative, launched in 2011, is a public-private effort that uses loans and grants to develop and finance new grocery stores, farmers' markets, and other food retail outlets. Its goal is to eliminate food deserts within seven years.[10]

In another welcome use of governmental authority, new rules for the federal school lunch program were announced in January 2012. By doubling the amount of fruits and vegetables served in schools, emphasizing whole grains, requiring the use of low-fat milk, and limiting salt and harmful fats, the federal government has taken a meaningful health-promotion step.[11]

Other laws and regulations could go further. Some interesting research suggests that taxing sugar-sweetened beverages by one penny per ounce could reduce the calories consumed from these beverages by about 10 percent. With research linking soda and other sugar-sweetened beverages to obesity, this commonsense solution should be considered at every level of government, despite the inevitable industry objections.[12]

Such a tax has an added benefit: generating revenues that governments can use to promote healthy living initiatives. A federal penny-per-ounce tax could generate almost $15 billion in its first year. There is a precedent for this approach in the routine use of federal, state, and local taxes on tobacco. Emphasizing the goal of improving our children's health, and insisting that the revenue stream is dedicated exclusively to public health initiatives, is the surest way to generate public support for a new tax.

At the federal level, we should be considering restricting junk-food advertising on television, especially at times when children are most likely to be watching, as the American Academy of Pediatrics has urged. Despite its pledges to reduce the marketing of unhealthy beverages to young people, the food industry seems to be doing just the opposite. A study from the Yale Rudd Center for Food Policy and Obesity found that youths viewed twice as many television ads for full-calorie soft drinks in 2010 than in 2008.[13]

Given how receptive children are to television advertising, we should be giving them age-appropriate messages that promote health, rather than undermine it. We should be conveying the enjoyment of eating healthy food, not sugary breakfast cereals and fast-food meals.

One reason so much high-fat, high-sugar food is sold so cheaply in the United States is the system of federal subsidies for commodity crops, mostly corn and soybeans. According to the California Public Interest Group (CalPIRG), taxpayers paid nearly $17 billion between 1995 and 2010 to subsidize four additives: corn syrup, high-fructose corn syrup, cornstarch, and soy oils.

A growing body of evidence suggests that high-fructose corn syrup, widely used in beverages, cereals, baked goods, and many other processed foods, may be harmful to our health. For one thing, it may generate stronger reward signals in our brains than glucose, prompting us to eat more fructose-sweetened products.[14] We also have research showing that animals that consumed high-fructose corn syrup gained more weight and were more likely to develop metabolic syndrome than animals that consumed the same number of calories in table sugar.[15] Metabolic syndrome, which is characterized by a cluster of symptoms that include excess body fat, high blood pressure, and high blood sugar, increases the risk of cancer, as well as of cardiovascular disease and diabetes.

A *Cancer Research* article described a more direct link, based on a laboratory finding that fructose can stimulate the proliferation of pancreatic cancer cells. The capacity of cancer cells to metabolize fructose to their benefit has "major significance for cancer patients," claimed the authors, who suggest that reducing fructose intake "may disrupt cancer growth."[16]

The 15-year, $17 billion subsidy for three corn-based additives and soy oils is enough "to buy each taxpayer 19 Twinkies" every year, according to CalPIRG. In the same period, taxpayers spent just $262 million subsidizing apples, the only fresh fruit that receives a significant federal subsidy. That translates into one-quarter of a Red Delicious apple per taxpayer.[17]

If we are looking for a dramatic example of misplaced priorities, we can certainly point to that one.

KEEPING AN EYE ON THE MARKETPLACE

In the industrial American food system, there is no predicting what will appear next on the grocery store shelves, or what risks it might carry. We do know that it is crucial to remain vigilant about what goes into our food, to monitor new production techniques as they are developed, and to raise our voices when threats to our health surface.

That's what happened when the dangers of trans fat, which come from partially hydrogenated vegetable oil, became apparent. The story demonstrates the power of bringing science, government, and advocacy together to strengthen public health and reduce the risk of cancer. Together, they generated a major change in the food system, although it came slowly, which is why I cannot say often enough that shifting toward an emphasis on prevention needs to begin now.

Trans fat, widely used in baked goods and deep-fried foods since the early 20th century, helps to prolong shelf life, keeps pie crusts flaky, and gives foods a distinctive taste and texture.

Researchers began to find compelling evidence of an association between trans fat and heart disease in the 1990s; the link to cancer emerged somewhat later. In 2006, Harvard researchers described an elevated risk of prostate cancer among men with higher levels of trans fat in their blood.[18] Two years later, the *American Journal of Epidemiology* published a study that found that French women who had higher blood levels of trans fat—"presumably reflecting a high intake of industrially processed foods"—were at least 50 percent more likely to have invasive breast cancer.[19]

As the evidence of health risks mounted, consumers took notice. In 1993, the Center for Science in the Public Interest (CSPI), a consumer watchdog group, asked the FDA to compel companies to disclose how much trans fat they used in their products.[20] Another decade passed before the FDA issued a final rule requiring trans fat to be listed on nutritional labels—and then gave manufacturers three years to comply. Since no level of trans fat is considered safe, one disappointing feature of the current law is that the label can list a product's trans fat content as zero if it contains less than one-half (0.5) of a gram.

Meanwhile, science moved forward, and the Institute of Medicine concluded in 2003 that it was feasible to exclude all trans fat derived from partially hydrogenated vegetable oil from food. In 2010, California became the first state to prohibit trans fat in restaurants, and many local governments have also issued bans. New York City, Boston, and Philadelphia all prohibit its use, as do counties in Massachusetts, New York, Pennsylvania, Washington State, and elsewhere. As the momentum for restrictions intensified, some chain restaurants switched to other fats, and food manufacturers began reformulating their products, substituting palm or hydrogenated oils for partially hydrogenated oil.

Still, trans fat remains on grocery store shelves in many locales, and just 18 percent of the American population lives in places where its use is banned in restaurants, according to the CSPI.[21] The CSPI and the American Public Health Association are among those call-ing for an across-the-board ban on all trans fat in food.[22]

Advocates need to keep the pressure on, and more governments should outlaw this unhealthy fat, but the regulations have clearly had an impact. As the use of trans fat declines, measures of harmful fatty acids in the blood are falling, too. The CDC says that blood levels of trans fat dropped by 58 percent from 2000 to 2009.[23]

While trans fat is trickling out of the food supply, genetically modi-fied organisms (GMOs) are gaining ground. Although a link to can-cer has not been established, we will need to keep a watchful eye to determine whether they are increasing our risk.

GMOs have had changes made to their genetic structure to cul-tivate a particular characteristic, such as resistance to insects or drought. The modifications can change how cantaloupes and toma-toes ripen and how well soybeans resist herbicides.

In contrast to conventional plant breeding, which is done in the field, genetic modifications occur in the laboratory with much greater speed and precision. Most of the commercial soy, canola, sugar beets, and corn grown in the United States have been geneti-cally modified, according to the American Academy of Environ-mental Medicine, and these ingredients are making their way into many of our processed foods. Gradually, genetically modified whole fruits and vegetables are being developed as well, including more than half of the papayas from Hawaii and some 24,000 acres of US zucchini and yellow squash. Other sources of GMOs in the human diet include a variety of food additives and products from animals that have eaten genetically modified foods.[24]

Currently, foods using GMOs do not need to be identified as such in the United States. Regulators use a "substantial equivalence" standard to determine safety—if the composition and nutritional value of a food is substantially equivalent to an existing food, it is considered to be equally safe. This essentially means there are no differences in the regulatory standards being applied whether or not a food has been genetically modified. The Europeans have taken the lead on this issue with their requirement that the use of GMOs be disclosed on product labels.

The FDA does regulate genetically engineered animals, which must be approved before they can be sold, and it has issued guidelines for companies seeking to develop them.[25] None of these animals are for sale yet, although a biotech firm has requested approval for a genetically modified salmon that could reach market size in 18 months, half the time usually required.[26] Three consumer groups have asked the FDA to regulate the inserted gene as a food additive, which would subject it to a more rigorous standard of review. The FDA has said only that it is reviewing the company's application. Clearly, industry is interested in using the tools of biotechnology to alter the food supply, and their use is likely to grow.

According to the Academy of Environmental Medicine, animal studies have shown that GMOs can alter immune function, initiate metabolic and cellular changes, and generate an inflammatory response. "It is biologically plausible for genetically modified foods to cause adverse health effects in humans," says the academy, which has called for a moratorium on sales of these foods until they can be adequately tested.[27]

The industry disagrees, of course, but we simply can't trust predictable industry assurances about the safety of genetically engineered food. We should be expecting, instead, that the federal government, especially the FDA, the EPA, and the US Department of Agriculture, serve the public interest by dedicating the resources necessary to conduct more research. Health professionals should also step forward to insist that we monitor genetically modified foods more carefully.

THE CANCER-PREVENTION DIET

While many environmental exposures and man-made products threaten our good health and increase our cancer risk, there is a lot we can do to nourish ourselves and our loved ones. Eating fresh, whole foods is the best way to meet the intertwined goals of losing weight, maintaining good health, and keeping cancer at bay. Some extracts with special anticancer properties should also be incorporated into our daily diets. Here are some guidelines.

Eat more fruits and vegetables. We have all heard this before, but the importance of including a range of fresh and colorful produce cannot be overstated. "A diet rich in fruits and vegetables should be at the heart of cancer prevention efforts," says Steven Kelly Clinton, MD, PhD, leader of molecular carcinogenesis and chemoprevention at the Ohio State University Comprehensive Cancer Center. "Each food contributes a little bit to lowering your cancer risk, just as each instrument contributes to the music produced by a symphony."

Attempts to isolate the specific cancer-preventing components of food have been consistently disappointing, however. If we can't single out one compound, it is probably because the nutrients in healthy foods are working together in a synergistic way that we don't fully understand.

The American Institute for Cancer Research, a nonprofit organization that studies the link between cancer and diet, highlights the cancer-fighting properties of the following foods:

- **Berries,** especially strawberries and raspberries, have a phytochemical called ellagic acid, which has antioxidant properties and in laboratory studies has been shown to deactivate carcinogens and slow cell reproduction. Blueberries also pack a powerful antioxidant punch.

- **Cruciferous vegetables,** including broccoli, brussels sprouts, cabbage, cauliflower, and broccoli rabe, are classified together by the four-petal flowers they sprout, which resemble a cross. These vegetables contain a heady number of health-promoting, cancer-fighting compounds, including isothiocyanates, indole-3-carbinol, glucosinolates, and sulforaphanes. These may be particularly helpful in reducing some of the cancers most associated with smoking, says Dr. Clinton. A presentation at a 2012 meeting of the American Institute for Cancer Research also suggested that cruciferous vegetables may increase survival among women who have had breast cancer.[28]

- **Tomatoes** are a potent source of lycopene, an antioxidant that gives them color and may be responsible for their anticancer benefits. Animal studies show that tomatoes reduce rates of prostate cancer, especially when they are used in processed or cooked form, such as tomato sauce. Laboratory studies also show that they can stop the growth of breast, lung, and endometrial cancer cells.

- **Dark green, leafy vegetables,** including kale, spinach, romaine lettuce, collard greens, and chard, are excellent sources of carotenoids, which have proven anticarcinogenic activity. Their powerful biological properties appear to give them a role in reducing the risk of oral cancers and cancers of the pancreas and colon. They also seem to inhibit the growth of breast, skin, lung, stomach, and other cancer cells, at least in the laboratory.

Buy organic. Fourteen hundred pesticides are approved for use by the EPA, and the President's Cancer Panel says human exposure to some of these products is linked to at least nine different cancers, including cancer of the breast, colon, lung, ovaries, pancreas, kidneys, and stomach.[29] The International Agency for Research on Cancer (IARC) classifies more than 400 chemicals, including those used in pesticides, as carcinogens or probable or possible carcinogens.[30]

Given how little we know about the cumulative impact of various chemical combinations, it makes sense to buy foods bearing the USDA-certified organic label whenever possible. An additional benefit is that most organic foods do not contain GMOs.

Eat more fiber. We have strong evidence that eating more fiber and more whole grains results in a reduced risk of colorectal cancer, according to a review of 25 studies published in the *British Medical Journal*. Fiber may dilute the carcinogens in the colon, reduce the time in which they remain there, enhance antioxidant action, or produce bacteria that promotes a healthy digestive tract.[31]

Researchers concluded that every 10 grams of daily fiber intake reduces the colon cancer risk by 10 percent. Good sources include whole grains, fruits, and vegetables. For example, a cup of cooked brown rice has 3.5 grams of fiber, a cup of blackberries almost

8 grams, and a cup of baked beans a little over 10 grams. You should aim for at least 25 grams per day.[32]

Eat more fish. Many are low in saturated fat and high in omega-3 fatty acids, including salmon, Atlantic mackerel, Arctic char, and sardines. We know for sure that these fish lower the risk of stroke and heart attack and reduce inflammation, which has been linked to the development of cancer. Fewer studies have looked directly at their role in preventing cancer, but some of the evidence is promising.

One study, reported in the *American Journal of Clinical Nutrition,* showed that fatty fish can reduce the risk of cancer of the oral cavity and pharynx, esophagus, stomach, colon and rectum, and pancreas.[33] Another found that women who ate fish rich in omega-3 fatty acids lowered their risk for colon polyps by about one-third. They also had lower levels of a hormone that can cause inflammation. (For reasons that were not clear, men enrolled in the study did not lower their risk for polyps.)[34]

Drink green tea. Green tea contains catechins, powerful antioxidants that are members of a class of compounds known as polyphenols, which may be able to protect cells from DNA damage. These polyphenols may also strengthen the immune system and activate enzymes that protect against tumor development.[35]

Although the NCI says the strength of the evidence is "not sufficient" to recommend the use of tea to prevent cancer, no one suggests there is any danger in consuming moderate amounts of it. Considering the promising laboratory findings, and the long tea-drinking tradition of Asian people, who tend to have lower rates of many types of cancer, drinking green tea is a healthy choice.

Increase your resveratrol. Resveratrol, found in red wine, red grapes, and peanuts, is another polyphenol that looks promising in animal studies. Its anti-inflammatory properties and its capacity to influence cell growth may explain how it helps to prevent cancer, although more research is needed to understand this fully.

We also don't know how much resveratrol it takes to gain meaningful protection. It makes sense to eat resveratrol-rich foods, but we would have to drink an unacceptable amount of red wine to benefit from it, especially given the link between alcohol and cancer.[36] We don't yet know much about the value of supplements.

Flavor your food with turmeric. This Indian spice, which gives curry its distinctly yellow color, contains the polyphenol curcumin. Hundreds of published papers over the past three decades have studied the antioxidant, anti-inflammatory, and preventive and therapeutic properties of curcumin, according to United Kingdom researchers writing in the *European Journal of Cancer*.[37] Ongoing research includes an NCI-funded study to assess curcumin's value in preventing abnormalities in the colon that may represent the early stages of colon polyps.[38]

Again, we can't say how much curcumin might help prevent cancer, or whether supplements have value, but turmeric is a flavorful and healthy addition to grains, fish, and vegetables.

Avoid red meat. A growing body of evidence points to an association between beef, pork, lamb, and goat and cancers of the colon, prostate, pancreas, and kidney. Researchers who followed more than 120,000 men and women for up to 28 years reported in the *Archives of Internal Medicine* that a daily serving of unprocessed red meat raising the odds of death from cancer by about 10 percent.[39] Processed meat, such as hot dogs, bacon and lunch meats, were worse, increasing the risk of cancer deaths by 17 percent. (Risk levels were even higher for heart disease.)

The link with colorectal cancer is especially strong, according to the American Institute for Cancer Research. That group says we can safely eat up to 18 ounces of red meat a week without increasing the cancer danger, but emphasizes the risk of consuming processed meats in any quantity.[40] Likewise, a series of studies involving almost half a million people indicated that those who ate 5 ounces or more of red meat a day were about one-third more likely to develop colon cancer, compared with those who consumed less than 1 ounce daily.[41]

There are a number of plausible reasons for this.[42] One theory is that the heme iron in meat, which gives it a red color, may damage the lining of the colon. Another is that a diet with too much red meat simply leaves less space for more nutritious, cancer-preventing foods. Carcinogens may also be present in smoked, salted, or cured meats and in meats cooked at high temperatures.

Limit alcohol consumption. Alcohol is a well-established risk factor for oral cancers; cancers of the esophagus, liver, colon, and breast; and possibly pancreatic cancer. Damage to cellular DNA may occur as the body metabolizes alcohol, and the link to breast cancer may be explained by a rise in estrogen levels in the blood. The American Cancer Society recommends that women have no more than one alcoholic drink daily and men no more than two (a single drink is defined as 12 ounces of beer, 5 ounces of wine, or 1.5 ounces of distilled spirits).

Limit processed foods. In *Food Rules: An Eater's Manual,* author Michael Pollan urges us to avoid any food with more than five ingredients or with ingredients we can't pronounce. That's a shorthand way of reminding us not to eat foods dominated by preservatives, additives, and ingredients that can't be found in nature. It's also a good way to avoid health-damaging trans fat and high-fructose corn syrup, which remain common in processed foods.

More research about what's harmful and helpful in the foods we eat is urgently needed. We should learn more about the risks of GMOs and have a better understanding of the nutrients that help prevent cancer. The National Cancer Institute, the American Cancer Society, the Institute of Medicine, and other agencies concerned about these issues should move forward now to guide us.

It will also be exciting to watch the results of ongoing studies examining anticancer agents in food sources.[43] Researchers at the University of Texas, Austin, are studying a plant lignin called SDG (secoisolariciresinol diglucoside), the active component of flaxseed, to see whether it can prevent breast cancer in premenopausal women who are at high risk. Columbia University scientists have pinpointed compounds in garlic that promote cell death and are studying an extract from green tea, called Poly E (polyphenon E), that might help prevent esophageal cancer.

At the same time, we already have plenty of knowledge about the individual behaviors and public policies that make a difference. The need to keep learning is no excuse not to take action today.

CHAPTER 13

THE POWER OF VITAMIN D

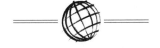

OMPELLING SCIENTIFIC RESEARCH HAS PER-suaded me that vitamin D is a valuable cancer-preventing agent, and I would like to see government and the medical community do more to promote its benefits. Some 3,000 published studies have investigated the association between vitamin D and cancer. After reviewing portions of that literature, researchers wrote in the *Annals of Epidemiology* that higher blood levels of vitamin D "are associated with substantially lower incidence rates of colon, breast, ovarian, renal, pancreatic, and aggressive prostate cancers."[1] Other cancers belong on that list as well, and *Principles and Practice of Oncology,* the classic oncology textbook, calls vitamin D "one of the most promising agents in cancer prevention research."[2]

The first randomized, placebo-controlled trial to assess the role that vitamin D and calcium play in cancer risk showed particularly convincing results. It was a gold-standard study design that followed almost 1,200 healthy postmenopausal women for four years. Researchers reported in the *American Journal of Clinical Nutrition* that women who took vitamin D plus calcium lowered their risk of developing any kind of cancer by 60 to 75 percent.[3]

"The evidence is strong enough to act on," says Dr. Robert P. Heaney, the John A. Creighton University Professor at Creighton University School of Medicine in Omaha, who is a leading expert on calcium and vitamin D. "The major vitamin D researchers share that opinion."

Based on what the science demonstrates, I think everyone should have their vitamin D blood levels measured and then discuss supplements with their doctors. A 2,000 IU daily dose of vitamin D is safe for most adults. When it is combined with an age-appropriate calcium supplement—generally, about 1,000 to 1,200 milligrams daily—it will in all likelihood decrease your cancer risk.

UNDERSTANDING VITAMIN D

Vitamin D is a *prohormone,* a precursor to a hormone with some of the same effects. Like other hormones, vitamin D influences cell function by binding to receptors in the cell membrane. It also plays a role in reducing inflammation and modulating the immune system.

Vitamin D's best-known role is to help us absorb calcium and maintain bone strength. We need it throughout our lives—as children to prevent rickets, characterized by soft, weak bones and skeletal deformities; and as adults to avoid osteomalacia, or soft bones, and osteoporosis, the brittle bone disease that is most common among the elderly.

Ten different mechanisms have been identified in the published literature to explain how vitamin D may work against cancer, and yet the link has still not received the attention it deserves.[4] Among the processes involved, vitamin D puts the brakes on the out-of-control division that is a hallmark of cancer cells and increases the expression of a gluelike substance called E-cadherin, which causes cells to stick together, inhibiting cancer invasion and metastasis. Vitamin D also promotes cell death and has anti-inflammatory activity. Other mechanisms include preventing the formation of blood vessels that feed cancer cells; interfering with signaling pathways that are active in certain cancers; and increasing the activity of tumor suppressor genes.

Vitamin D has other benefits as well. Research indicates that higher levels of vitamin D in the blood may lower the risk for heart disease, high blood pressure, diabetes, multiple sclerosis, and Parkinson's disease, assuming there's also an adequate level of calcium.

Sunlight triggers the production of vitamin D in the skin, and relatively short exposures raise vitamin D levels significantly. Some researchers suggest spending 5 to 30 minutes in the sun between 10 a.m. and 3 p.m. at least twice a week, although that conflicts with concerns about protecting the skin at all times to avoid skin cancer. Moreover, in northern climes, the angle of the sun from November to April makes it difficult to absorb the UVB rays necessary for adequate vitamin D synthesis. Cloud cover, smog, the melanin content of the skin, and the use of sunscreen further limit the amount of vitamin D our bodies are able to manufacture.

It is also difficult to get enough vitamin D from food, although dietary contributions can help. Much of the vitamin D in the American diet comes from fortified foods, primarily milk, but it is also added to some yogurts, juices, and breakfast cereals. Cod and salmon are especially high in vitamin D, and tuna, mackerel, and sardines contain meaningful amounts as well. Old-fashioned though it may sound, a tablespoon of cod liver oil is another great source.

To raise vitamin D blood levels, most of us will need to take supplements. Vitamin D comes in two forms: D_2 (ergocalciferol) and D_3 (cholecalciferol). Fortified foods and supplements can contain either form, while sunlight exposure produces D_3. Although equivalent in many ways, vitamin D_3 is more potent and the form many experts prefer.

Vitamin D is metabolized in our bodies in a series of steps. First, it is converted in the liver to calcidiol—the chemical name is 25-hydroxyvitamin D, or 25(OH)D—and then the kidneys take action, forming calcitriol. A physician needs to measure the level of calcidiol in your blood to determine your vitamin D status.

Levels of vitamin D in the blood are expressed in two ways: as either nanomoles per liter of blood (nmol/l) or nanograms per milliliter of blood (ng/ml). According to the Institute of Medicine (IOM), a person is deficient in vitamin D if his or her level falls below 30 nmol/l (12 ng/ml), at which point rickets or osteomalacia typically occur. Vitamin D levels in the blood between 30 and 50 nmol/l (12 to 20 ng/ml) are also considered inadequate for bone and overall health. The IOM generally considers a vitamin D measure at or above 50 nmol/l (20 ng/ml) adequate for good health.

There is considerable disagreement about the level that creates a health risk. The IOM says the potential for adverse effects—such as kidney stones and kidney damage—can occur when vitamin D levels rise above 125 nmol/l (50 ng/ml). The Vitamin D Council, on the other hand, states that the vitamin D toxicity level is 500 to

750 nmol/l (200 to 250 ng/ml), with a safe upper limit of 250 nmol/l, or 100 ng/ml.

The IOM does not address the dose of vitamin D that is effective for cancer prevention. Many vitamin D experts recommend between 100 and 150 nmol/l (40 and 60 ng/ml) for that purpose.

A BODY OF EVIDENCE DEVELOPS

A link between cancer and sunlight was first suspected back in 1936, when a physician noticed that US Navy personnel who had been diagnosed with skin cancer—presumably suggesting excess exposure to the sun—developed fewer cancers in other locations of the body. A few years later, a researcher reported that cancer death rates were lower in parts of the United States that received more sunlight.[5] In those days, the explanation for these relationships was not well understood.

In 1970, the National Cancer Institute (NCI) published maps of the incidence of cancer and cancer deaths in the United States. Cedric Garland, DrPH, and his brother, Frank Garland, PhD, then both public health specialists and epidemiologists at the Johns Hopkins School of Public Health, noticed that people in the northern parts of the country were more likely to die from colorectal cancer than people who lived in the South.

Intrigued, the Garlands began an investigation, and in 1980 they published an article in the *International Journal of Epidemiology* suggesting that vitamin D and calcium work together to provide protection against colon cancer.[6]

A subsequent study of almost 2,000 men who had been followed for 19 years supported that theory—as reported in the *Lancet,* the greater the intake of vitamin D and calcium, the lower the colon cancer risk.[7]

The case for vitamin D continued to build. In the *Journal of the National Cancer Institute*, researchers described a link between vitamin D levels and a reduced risk of the colon polyps that have the potential to become malignant.[8]

Likewise, pooled results from five studies found a dramatically lowered colon cancer risk among people with higher levels of vitamin D in their blood, according to the *American Journal of Preventive Medicine*. Data from almost 1,500 people who had been followed for 25 years showed that those whose vitamin D blood levels measured 33 ng/ml or higher had a 50 percent lower risk of developing colon cancer than those whose vitamin D levels measured 12 ng/ml or below.[9]

The protective effect of vitamin D against breast cancer has also been well documented, with women who have the highest levels of vitamin D in their blood consistently showing the lowest risk of developing breast cancer.[10] The randomized, placebo-controlled trial conducted at the Osteoporosis Research Center at Creighton University was designed to raise circulating vitamin D levels in the study group to 80 nmol/l, which is the higher end of the "adequate" range. After four years, the study found that about 3 percent of women given 1,100 IU of vitamin D plus a calcium supplement developed cancer. By contrast, nearly 4 percent of those taking calcium alone, and 7 percent of those taking a placebo, developed cancer.

Because these kinds of results have been slow to influence behavior, it is worth highlighting a few other studies to demonstrate the consistent strength of the findings. One analysis, published in the *American Journal of Clinical Nutrition*, drew on data from the Women's Health Initiative (one of the largest prevention studies ever conducted in the United States).[11] It found that women who took vitamin D and calcium supplements (400 IU of vitamin D and 1,000 milligrams of calcium) for seven years decreased their risk of any form of cancer, of breast cancer, and of invasive breast cancer by an average of 14 to 20 percent.

Another study, appearing in the *Journal of Steroid Biochemistry and Molecular Biology*, reported that women with blood levels of vitamin D less than 13 ng/ml had the highest risk of breast cancer, while those whose vitamin D blood levels were approximately 52 ng/ml had the lowest risk. The researchers report that 2,000 IU of vitamin D_3 daily and very moderate exposure to sunlight, about 12 minutes per day, could reduce breast cancer incidence by 50 percent.[12]

LOST OPPORTUNITIES

Given these and other impressive findings, it is puzzling that our government and public health officials aren't actively encouraging people to increase their vitamin D intake.

In 2010, the IOM revised its recommended Dietary Reference Intakes (DRIs) for calcium and vitamin D. Formulated by physicians, scientists, and epidemiologists, DRIs are guidelines to the daily intake of nutrients considered sufficient to meet the health requirements of most Americans. New vitamin D recommendations had been eagerly awaited by experts who felt that the existing ones— 200 IU for people ages 1 through 50; 400 IU for ages 51 to 70; and 600 IU for those over 70—were far too low.

Many vitamin D enthusiasts were disappointed when the IOM raised the recommended dosage only slightly: to 600 IU per day for people ages 1 to 70 and to 800 IU per day for those over 70. The

IOM increased calcium DRIs at the same time, recommending 1,000 milligrams for adults ages 19 to 50 and 1,200 milligrams for women 51 to 70.

Yet the IOM acknowledges that 4,000 IU of vitamin D daily is safe for people ages 9 to 70, including pregnant and lactating women. Exceed that, and the IOM says the risk of being harmed increases, although it has also indicated that "no observed adverse effect" has been identified at levels as high as 10,000 IU.

The small increases in the new guidelines generated an outpouring of criticism from the medical community. Based on an analysis of vitamin D's impact on bone health, the *Harvard School of Public Health Nutrition Source* claimed that the IOM's threshold was not supported by the available data.[13] The International Osteoporosis Foundation recommended 800 to 1,000 IU of vitamin D for anyone age 60 or older.[14]

"The Institute of Medicine recommendations are defective," Dr. Heaney says. "They aren't enough. The IOM committee didn't do its job adequately."

A letter of consensus, signed by 40 leading vitamin D experts around the world—including Dr. Heaney and Dr. Cedric Garland, who is now a professor of family and preventive medicine at the University of California, San Diego, School of Medicine—calls for people to maintain vitamin D blood levels of between 40 and 60 ng/ml to prevent a host of diseases, including osteoporosis, certain cancers, diabetes, and heart failure. The experts call for a "nearly universal oral intake of vitamin D_3 of 2,000 IU/day."[15]

In *Current Opinion in Clinical Nutrition and Metabolic Care*, Dr. Heaney writes, "It is useful to note that there are effectively no recorded cases of vitamin D intoxication at serum 25(OH)D levels below 350 nmol/l. Given that fact, it seems both safe and prudent to state that serum 25(OH)D values between 120 and 225 nmol/l demarcate the normal range."[16] According to Dr. Heaney, the burden of proof lies with those who dispute the need for higher doses of vitamin D.

———

Unfortunately, design flaws could undermine the one major study that might produce data definitive enough to compel the federal government to issue a more appropriate recommendation about vitamin D's broader role in health.

The Vitamin D and Omega-3 Trial, known as the VITAL Study,[17] is funded by the National Institutes of Health and will investigate the effects of vitamin D and fish oil supplements on the risk of cancer, heart disease, and stroke. This study is being conducted by researchers from Harvard Medical School, School of Public Health and Brigham and Women's Hospital in Boston.

The 20,000-person study will divide participants into four groups. One group will take 2,000 IU of vitamin D per day, plus 1,000 milligrams of fish oil, and another will take two placebos. The two other groups will take one active nutrient and one placebo apiece—either vitamin D and a fish oil placebo or a vitamin D placebo and fish oil.

Unfortuntely, there are several problems inherent in the VITAL Study. First, vitamin D blood levels are not being measured from the start, so researchers won't know who has deficient or adequate levels. Second, with the increased interest in vitamin D, some people are likely to take the supplement on their own, which is permitted, making it more difficult to pinpoint the vitamin's effect.

Finally, and perhaps of greatest concern, calcium is not included in the study. "Calcium and vitamin D work together," says Dr. Cedric Garland. "It's unnatural to separate them. Even if calcium weren't essential to cancer prevention, giving calcium with vitamin D is the only way to promote good bone health."

Despite the time, money, and resources being dedicated to the VITAL study, many vitamin D experts believe it is designed to fail. "There is a strong probability that the study will be inconclusive," Dr. Heaney says.

Taking Action Now

Whatever the limitations and findings of the VITAL study, many scientists believe we have enough evidence that vitamin D plays a role in overall health and cancer prevention—and many of them are acting on their own conviction. "A few years ago, the CDC convened a panel to develop optimal vitamin D supplements for elderly, institutionalized people," Dr. Heaney recalls. "As part of that group, I asked my colleagues, consisting of vitamin D scientists, how much vitamin D they themselves were taking per day. Everyone in that room was taking 5,500 IU per day. Nearly all vitamin D scientists have come to the same conclusion."

In 2007, breast cancer survivor and Grassroots Health founder Carole Baggerly attended a NCI–sponsored conference focused on vitamin D and cancer. "I was stunned by the body of evidence in support of D's role in cancer prevention," she says, recalling the presentations.

Almost as stunning to her was the litany repeated by panelists as they were asked about the next steps. "We need more research," they kept saying.

Baggerly felt disappointed and frustrated. "I don't challenge the need for more research, but after listening for a while, I felt compelled to speak. I stood up and asked, 'Where is your sense of urgency?'"

She says that when the meeting ended, one scientist after another approached her to talk further. "They asked me, 'How can we help you get the message out?' Every one of them was passionate about their work, but they didn't have a vehicle." Soon afterward, she and her husband founded GrassrootsHealth, dedicated to eliminating vitamin D deficiencies around the world.

Enlightened by the evidence, my family and I have our doctors test our vitamin D levels at least once a year, and we all take a vitamin D supplement, in addition to a daily multivitamin that contains calcium.

The appropriate supplement dose depends on each person's level of vitamin D in the bloodstream. That's why your doctor should first measure your vitamin D level and then discuss the supplement dose that is right for you. This is a personalized approach to vitamin D supplementation that is safe and effective.

In my home, we don't expect our vitamin D intake to substitute for other healthy practices. As Dr. Heaney says, "nutrients are not solo players, but rather ensemble players. They all work together." I also serve my family healthful meals, rich in a variety of vegetables, fruits, and whole grains, with a minimal amount of red meat.

I know that taking vitamin D supplements hasn't harmed us, and we have good reason to believe that it is decreasing our cancer risk.

CHAPTER 14

CAN PILLS PREVENT CANCER?

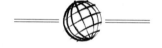

MOST PEOPLE WOULD LIKE TO FIND A MAGIC bullet to reduce the risk of cancer or prevent its recurrence, which is why chemoprevention—the use of drugs, vitamins, and other agents—holds tremendous appeal. Unfortunately, with the exception of vitamin D, our current chemopreventive agents have significant risks along with their benefits.

While we do have some therapies that may be useful for people who have already had cancer, or for people at high risk for it, using potent medications as agents of cancer prevention in large populations of healthy people has to meet higher standards of safety and effectiveness. Right now, we don't know enough to recommend their broad use.

That's not what the pharmaceutical companies would like you to think. They have always been good at marketing powerful drugs for long-term use by a large number of people, because that's how they make their biggest profits. A generation of women took hormone replacement therapy not only to ease the symptoms of menopause but also because of the promise that it would reduce their risk of heart disease and offer other health benefits. Instead, studies showed that combined (estrogen and progestin) hormone therapy significantly *increased* the risk of death from breast cancer. Women who took either combined hormone therapy or estrogen alone had a higher risk of stroke, blood clots, and heart attack, and their mammograms were more difficult to evaluate because of the hormonal stimulation.

For now, vitamin D with calcium is the only chemopreventive measure I can recommend wholeheartedly for healthy people. Here is what you should know about some of the other agents being promoted for the prevention of cancer.

Aspirin and Other Nonsteroidal Anti-Inflammatory Drugs

We have known something about the anticancer properties of nonsteroidal anti-inflammatory drugs (NSAIDs) since the 1970s. Various studies have shown that aspirin and other NSAIDs can suppress the development of some potentially malignant polyps, prevent polyps from recurring in people who have had them previously, cause existing polyps to regress, and reduce death rates from colorectal cancer.

In one study, researchers looked at the aspirin use of almost 83,000 women who had provided information about their medication history from 1980 to 2000 as part of the Nurses' Health Study.

The researchers wrote in the *Journal of the American Medical Association* that aspirin did reduce the risk of colon cancer significantly, but it took 10 years of regular use to do it. The biggest risk reduction came with the use of more than 14 aspirin tablets a week.[1]

A review of eight other studies, published in the *Lancet,* went further. After five years of taking aspirin, participants had lower death rates from esophageal, pancreatic, brain, and lung cancer. Death rates from stomach, colorectal, and prostate cancer fell as well, but required longer periods of aspirin use.[2]

My reluctance to recommend aspirin enthusiastically for everyone stems from its side effects. The *Journal of the American Medical Association* study confirmed that the aspirin-associated risk of gastrointestinal bleeding rises with increasing doses of the drug. We also know that hemorrhagic stroke is a rare but possible side effect of aspirin. If more people take aspirin at higher doses for longer periods of time, we will probably see more of that.

For those reasons, I don't advise people to take aspirin if they are doing so only in the hopes of preventing cancer. I am, however, comfortable with the perspective offered by Andrew Dannenberg, MD, professor of medicine and director of Cancer Prevention at Weill Medical College of Cornell University in New York City. He says, "If your cardiologist recommends taking aspirin for cardiovascular disease protection, there may be secondary benefits, such as the reduced risk of colon cancer."

Statins

Statins, the widely used medications to lower cholesterol levels, may also help control the initiation and growth of tumors, and possibly metastatic disease. According to an analysis published in the

New England Journal of Medicine, statins were associated with a 47 percent drop in the relative risk of colorectal cancer.[3] Where a population would ordinarily have about 42 cases of colorectal cancer per 100,000 people, at least five years of statin use might prevent almost half of those cases.

Impressive though this sounds, it means that in a population with an average risk of colon cancer, more than 4,800 people would have to be treated to prevent a single case. While a reduced cancer risk may be a welcome side effect of treating high cholesterol, that kind of statistic raises serious questions about the use of statins for cancer prevention in people with normal cholesterol levels. That's especially so given the potential side effects. In February 2011, the FDA announced that almost a dozen commonly used statins can cause liver toxicity, memory loss and confusion, muscle damage, and increases in blood sugar that could lead to type 2 diabetes.

So far, statins do not seem to have much value in preventing other cancers, at least after short-term use. As reported in the *European Journal of Cancer,* a systematic analysis of 42 studies found that statins had no effect on the overall incidence of cancer, or on the incidence of lung, breast, or prostate cancer. They do seem to offer some protection from stomach and liver cancer, but may actually be associated with an increase in melanoma and non-melanoma skin cancer. Most of the evidence is weak, the study's authors wrote, and more studies with a longer follow-up are needed.[4]

METFORMIN

In animal studies, metformin, a drug used to treat type-2 diabetes, appears to make cancers less aggressive.[5] Scientists are looking more closely at its possible role in preventing colorectal, breast, pancreatic, liver, and prostate cancers, though the research is in its early stages.[6]

Again, there are concerns about side effects. Metformin can cause lactic acidosis, a condition that occurs when lactic acid accumulates in the bloodstream faster than it can be removed. Lactic acid is produced when oxygen levels in the body decrease. Although the risk is of lactic acidosis is low, the condition can be fatal. It is enough of a concern to warrant the advice that patients taking metformin have their electrolyte levels carefully monitored. This risk limits the widespread use of metformin for cancer prevention.

HORMONAL THERAPIES

Two classes of hormonal therapies—selective estrogen receptor modulators, such as tamoxifen and raloxifene, and aromatase inhibitors—are currently approved by the FDA as adjuvant therapy to prevent a recurrence among women who have been treated for breast cancer.

In 2006, after the STAR (Study of Tamoxifen and Raloxifene) trial demonstrated that tamoxifen and raloxifene could reduce the likelihood of invasive breast cancer in high-risk healthy women—by 50 percent for tamoxifen and 38 percent for raloxifene—more oncologists began prescribing them.[7] However, once again, their side effects—including an elevated risk of endometrial cancer and blood clots—limit their value, so their use as chemopreventive agents is not recommended for average-risk women. The risk of uterine cancer and blood clots is higher with tamoxifen than with raloxifene.

An ongoing study, called the MAP.3 trial, sponsored by the National Cancer Institute of Canada, is evaluating the possible role of one aromatase inhibitor, exemestane, in cancer prevention among 4,560 high-risk women. A preliminary analysis at three years of follow-up found that the drug reduced the incidence of invasive breast cancer by 65 percent and also lowered the odds of ductal carcinoma in situ (DCIS). In women who did develop invasive cancer, the tumors were less aggressive than those that occurred in women in the placebo group. These promising early results led researchers to close the placebo arm so that all participants could have the choice to take exemestane.[8]

Despite that good news, side effects of exemestane, especially extreme joint pain and menopausal symptoms such as hot flashes, caused approximately 10 percent of patients per year in the study to stop taking the drug.[9] A separate study, published in *Lancet Oncology*, evaluated the bone health of a subgroup of women participating in the MAP.3 trial.[10] Researchers found that the women taking daily exemestane had a greater decline in bone mineral density after two years of treatment than the women taking the placebo. Additional follow-up is necessary to determine whether women taking exemestane have a higher risk of bone fracture. We already know that prolonged use of aromatase inhibitors can cause heart disease and osteoporosis, again suggesting they will have limited value in healthy women.

There are enough uncertainties and risks associated with the available chemopreventive agents to serve as a warning to us all. Nonetheless, I remain optimistic that this will eventually prove to be a fruitful area of research. Work in that field continues across the country and should be intensified.

CHAPTER 15

ON THE CUTTING EDGE OF SCIENCE

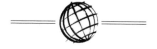

SHREE BOSE WAS A 17-YEAR-OLD HIGH SCHOOL junior in Fort Worth, Texas, when she won the grand prize in the inaugural Google Global Science Fair, in 2011.

Bose was trying to understand why patients treated with cisplatin, a powerful chemotherapy drug used to treat ovarian cancer, often develop resistance to it. Under the supervision of Alakananda Basu, PhD, a professor of molecular biology and immunology at the University of North Texas Health Science Center, Bose studied adenosine monophosphate-activated protein kinase, a protein that is supposed to tell the cells when they can and cannot use energy to replicate. Her experiment established a link between the protein and a resistance to cisplatin, setting the stage for the development of techniques to enable the drug to retain its potency as a cancer killer.

I asked Bose where she had developed her passion for science and why she had chosen to spend her summer vacation sequestered in a hospital laboratory. Her answer was very personal: Her grandfather's death from liver cancer two years earlier had affected her deeply. "I decided that I wanted to enter cancer research, so that none of my other family members would have to suffer from cancer," she said. "It was very difficult to see what cancer did to this extremely active man."

Bose is headed to Harvard University in the fall of 2012 and hopes to pursue a career in science and research. In a Huffington Post blog, she highlighted two eye-opening insights that resulted from the Global Science Fair. One was her realization that scientists were not really "superhuman," but simply intelligent and hardworking. "That's the thing about science fairs," she wrote, "anyone with a good idea and the determination to work at it can win, and those are the people who are out there changing the world."

The other was that scientific advances truly change lives. "I now hear from people all around the country who have suffered from ovarian cancer or know people who have, and they thank me for my work. I think that's the feeling most researchers strive for their entire lives."[1]

Hopefully, Shree Bose will fulfill her dream of combining cancer research with medical practice, joining a new generation of scientists who will transform the cancer culture.

Thanks to the work of dedicated researchers like her, we have made meaningful progress, especially in our understanding of the biology of cancer. I've made it clear that I think we can do much better, and we can do it in a more focused, goal-oriented way, but here I want to commend some of the promising research that is under way, with funding from both public and private sources. As I see it, there are at least four avenues that merit further exploration: vaccines, microbes, the tumor microenvironment, and the human microbiome.

TAKING AIM AT CANCER THROUGH VACCINES

We already have vaccines to disable two cancer-causing viruses—the hepatitis B virus, which can cause liver cancer, and HPV, which can cause cervical and other types of cancer. These are traditional vaccines that work by introducing weakened or inactive forms of the virus into the body, jump-starting an immune response that prevents a viral invader from causing disease.

Scientists have also made some progress developing vaccines that can target and destroy cancer cells. In theory, this is what our bodies are already doing. Researchers believe that many of us—perhaps even most—have had cancer cells in our bodies at one time or another. Because the immune system quietly went about its business of killing or suppressing those aberrant cells before they could coalesce into a detectable tumor, we never even knew they were there. It is only when our immune systems fail at this task that cancer can flourish.

Just one vaccine has been approved to fight active cancer: sipuleucel-T (Provenge), used to treat metastatic prostate cancer.[2]

Licensed by the FDA in July 2010, it is about as controversial as any cancer therapy on the market. Approval was largely based on data demonstrating an improved median survival time of 4.1 months among men treated with the vaccine, although researchers suggested in the *Journal of the National Cancer Institute* that the actual survival benefit may be smaller.[3]

Of course, vaccine research has to start somewhere, and we should not be surprised by early disappointments. Still, we hope for more significant results, especially when such limited improvement comes at such an exorbitant price: $93,000 for treatment with Provenge, which doesn't include additional expenses to cover doctor visits and other needed care.[4]

Clearly, a larger number of more-effective vaccines and immune-based therapies are needed. Working at the forefront of tumor immunology, immunotherapy, and the interactions between tumor and immune system cells, 250 scientists and clinicians at the National Cancer Institute's (NCI) Laboratory of Tumor Immunology and Biology have made a commitment to try to develop such therapies. One of their objectives is to find points of vulnerability that are present only on tumor cells, not on normal cells.

"The immune system has the capability of specifically identifying the precise targets that may be found only on tumor cells, or over-expressed on tumor cells," explains James L. Gulley, MD, PhD, who directs the Clinical Trials Group at the NCI immunology lab. The goal is to use vaccines to help train the immune system to recognize and kill the cells that contain those markers. "We're not directly targeting the tumor with the vaccine. We're directly targeting the immune system, which then starts targeting the tumor."

For example, Dr. Gulley's team tested the pan-carcinoma vaccine (PANVAC)—which contains viruses that identify cancer cells, prompting the body's immune system to attack—on 26 patients with metastatic breast or ovarian cancers. A single patient, who had been diagnosed with breast cancer in her 30s and had metastatic disease by the time she enrolled in the trial, generated particular excitement among the researchers.[5] More than three years after she was vaccinated, her disease had not progressed and could not be detected on scans. "It's wonderful," says Dr. Gulley with guarded optimism. "I wish we would see this in every patient."

In her case, a number of clinical features offer guidance for future research. Despite the metastases, her cancer did not appear to have spread widely, and her last round of chemotherapy had been 12 months prior to enrolling in the trial, so her immune system was relatively strong. Significantly, the woman had also participated in a previous vaccine study, which may have helped to stimulate her immune system, increasing the second vaccine's effectiveness.

Researchers continue to investigate the best ways to use vaccines in conjunction with standard treatments to generate better outcomes. "We are making great headway in our ability to combine vaccines with standard therapies," Dr. Gulley claims. "We've combined a vaccine with chemotherapy, hormonal therapy, and radiation therapy and also small molecule inhibitors."

Custom-tailored treatment is on the horizon. Dr. Gulley expects that physicians will eventually be able to develop a profile of both patient and tumor to better help them decide, for example, that one person will benefit from a vaccine given after a single cycle of chemotherapy, while another will generate enough of an immune response from the vaccine to be able to avoid chemotherapy altogether. "We're going to have the information available so that in about 10 years there would be five or six vaccines available for various patients," he believes.

A number of vaccine trials are helping to build the necessary storehouse of knowledge. For example, a study found that patients with metastatic colorectal cancer who had received the standard treatment combined with an experimental vaccine survived longer than patients who had received only the standard treatment.[6] We also have some promising data about the value of vaccines for various kinds of lymphoma.

I am eagerly awaiting the results of a clinical trial launched by the NCI in January 2011 to test the effectiveness of a vaccine to treat glioblastoma multiforme, one of the deadliest brain cancers.[7] My childhood friend Oksana was diagnosed with that disease in her early 40s and died a few years later, after a long and difficult treatment. Oksana would so have wanted better treatment options, not only for herself but also for those who came after her.

An even better innovation would be a full complement of preventive vaccines that can be administered routinely to stop cells from ever turning cancerous.

"Prevention trials take a lot more patients to show an impact because most people won't get the disease, and those who do get the disease may not die from it," says Dr. Gulley. In other words, most people are going to die from causes other than those the vaccine is intended to prevent, so meaningful comparisons between vaccinated and nonvaccinated populations are impossible without large and costly studies. However, we know from our experience with other successful vaccines, including those for HPV, hepatitis B, smallpox, and polio, that it is possible to design clinical trials in a way that will obtain useful information in a reasonable amount of time. A collaborative effort focusing on the development of new cancer-preventing vaccines could yield remarkable results.

USING MICROBES TO DELIVER TREATMENT

Not all viruses are harmful; some can be engineered to treat or prevent cancer. These oncolytic viruses can be executed in two ways. In one design, the virus infects only cancer cells, where it replicates vigorously and destroys its hosts. In an alternative design, the virus can penetrate both cancer and normal cells, but its ability to reproduce and destroy is limited to cancer cells. In addition to attacking cancer cells, oncolytic viruses can be used as a therapy delivery system, carrying immune-boosting genes to galvanize the energies of white blood cells and other components of the immune system. *Vaccinia poxvirus,* the adapted virus that helped to eliminate smallpox, is now being tested as a potential cancer treatment, as are modified forms of the herpes virus and other pathogens.

The Lung Cancer Research Foundation (LCRF) is funding one study at the University of Louisville, Kentucky, in which researchers hope that a virus can deliver treatment with fewer side effects than traditional approaches.[8] At the University of Pittsburgh Cancer Institute, researchers funded by LCRF are conducting a clinical trial to evaluate the safety of the *vaccinia* virus in lung cancer patients.[9] Meanwhile, two National Cancer Institute studies are looking at the same virus for use in the treatment of liver cancer.[10]

There is also an LCRF-funded study using bacteria as a delivery device under way at the University of Minnesota. This one uses a deactivated form of salmonella, which can be a deadly food contaminant. With the toxic effects bioengineered out, the goal is to deliver immune system stimulants to kill lung cancer cells.[11]

Right now, microbes are being studied as treatment tools, not as a prevention strategy. They are generally more effective when paired with chemotherapy or radiation, which means we are a long way from being able to eliminate our standard toxic treatments. However, honing our ability to deliver targeted therapy is an important start in a new direction.

THE TUMOR MICROENVIRONMENT

Cancer cells do not live in a vacuum, but rather they rely on a complex system of normal cells, blood vessels, microscopic organisms, and molecules for nourishment and protection. Among the elements of this cooperative network are macrophages, which help to alert the rest of the immune system to the presence of invaders; and fibroblasts, the most common type of cell in connective tissue.

"More than 10 years ago, we began to understand that a tumor is like any other organ, in that it has vascular cells, immune cells, neurons, and fibroblasts," explains Suresh Mohla, PhD, who directs the Tumor Microenvironment Network at the NCI. "All of those cells have a role in the life of the tumor. As a tumor evolves, the microenvironment cells evolve as well."

The Tumor Microenvironment Network funds programs at 11 universities and medical centers. Researchers at MD Anderson Cancer Center are studying the framework that supports tumors and their ability to develop resistance to therapy. Meanwhile, a team at the Albert Einstein College of Medicine in New York is helping to identify subtypes of tumor macrophages and to delineate their role in promoting the growth of tumors and their capacity to metastasize.[12]

This research has led to discoveries that increase our capacity to exploit some of the microenvironment's features. We have already learned, for example, that cancer cells closest to the tumor function differently from those farther away, and that some nearby macrophages and fibroblasts develop the capacity to help a tumor progress. We also know that as soon as a tumor is formed, it sends signals to the bone marrow. The bone marrow then helps to suppress the immune cells so the tumor can continue to grow. "Cancer is like a foreign body. Normally, it would be rejected, but cancer cells fool the immune system by sending the message "I'm not your enemy; I'm your friend," says Mohla.

Tumor cells often lie dormant for decades before beginning to spread. "How do tumor cells live for 20 years in the bone marrow and then suddenly become active, allowing the cancer to metastasize?" asks Mohla. "If we understood the microenvironment of the dormant tumor, than we would have the means to make the active tumor go back to dormancy." With funding by the Sussman Family Fund for Breast Cancer Research, scientists at Memorial Sloan-Kettering are exploring that question as they try to identify the distinctive characteristics of dormant breast and prostate cancer cells.

THE HUMAN MICROBIOME PROJECT

The microorganisms that make their homes in our bodies outnumber human cells by an estimated 10 to 1. The complex ecosystem known as the human microbiome, with its many viruses, bacteria, and other microscopic forms of life, influences health and disease in ways we are only beginning to understand.

The Human Microbiome Project, launched in 2007 by the National Institutes of Health (NIH), is designed to inventory the microbes that live harmoniously in our bodies. The ultimate goal is to find ways to improve human health by monitoring or manipulating the microbiome.[13] Eventually that knowledge may allow us to take early and preemptive action. As NIH director Francis S. Collins writes in *The Language of Life*, ". . . it is not hard to imagine a time in the future when routine sampling of the microbiome from various body sites will be utilized as an early warning sign of trouble, even before symptoms have appeared."[14]

During the first phase of the Human Microbiome Project, funded for five years at a cost of $150 million, researchers sequenced the genes of hundreds of bacteria, most of them in five sites of the body—the gastrointestinal tract, the mouth, the vagina, the skin, and the nasal cavity. That work continues, with plans to sequence additional bacteria, viruses, and other microbes from a total of 18 body sites.

Meanwhile, demonstration projects studying the relationship between the human microbiome and health are in progress at universities across the country. One example in the cancer realm is a New York University School of Medicine study of bacteria native to the esophagus.[15] Researchers are testing their hypothesis that changes in the microbiome of the foregut, which runs from the mouth to the first part of the small intestine, are associated with a type of esophageal cancer that has jumped sixfold in the past 30 years. Among a study group of elderly male veterans, those who carried a specific microorganism called microbiota type II were at least 15 times more likely to develop precursors of esophageal cancer, including reflux esophagitis and Barrett's esophagus, compared with a similar population carrying microbiota type I.

Other studies may eventually tell us whether an abnormal microbiome plays a role in the development of esophageal carcinoma, and whether antibiotics or probiotics can help prevent it. The results could reverse the rise in esophageal cancer and offer lessons for fighting other types of cancer.

ADVANCING RESEARCH THROUGH PRIVATE FUNDING

Since scientific progress can take a long time, scientists need assurance that capital will be available to sustain their work over many years. In an interview conducted by the Ovarian Cancer Research Fund, Jonathan S. Berek, MD, a member of the fund's Scientific Advisory Committee, shared his views: "If you don't support people early in their careers, they will be attracted to enter other challenging fields that provide greater stability and resource. It's very Darwinian—it's the survival of not only the fittest but also the best funded. Scientists tend to pursue opportunities that can be sustained. As funding for research through our government has remained flat or decreased over the years, it becomes an extraordinary challenge to attract and retain the brightest and the best to conduct the cancer research that is so essential."[16]

That's where donations to private research foundations and advocacy groups come in. Some of the most exciting research is being funded by such organizations, and a few of the most impressive ones are highlighted below.

The Ovarian Cancer Research Fund, the largest independent organization in the United States dedicated exclusively to funding research into this disease, has awarded 164 grants totaling nearly $40 million to 62 leading medical centers since 1998. Among many other avenues of research, some of the work is aimed at early-stage detection, building knowledge about the underlying genetics and molecular biology of ovarian cancer, and finding ways to "super-charge" the immune response. The fund also supports the Cooperative Ovarian Cancer Group for Immunotherapy, based at Stanford University and headed by Dr. Berek. This consortium of ovarian cancer researchers from 29 top medical centers in the United States and the United Kingdom is committed to developing novel immunotherapies and vaccines.

The National Breast Cancer Coalition has created the Artemis Project to search for a preventive vaccine in conjunction with its Breast Cancer Deadline 2020 project. Four work groups are focused on key issues that need to be addressed to reach that goal: identifying the most appropriate targets of a vaccine; understanding how the immune system responds to breast cancer in order to know what the vaccine needs to accomplish; deciding when to offer a vaccine, and to whom; and making sure the vaccine is safe.

Writing on the Huffington Post, coalition president Fran Visco noted how scientific advances in immunology, genetics, vaccine technology, and elsewhere have "created an unprecedented opportunity for development of a preventive vaccine." She said, "We could not have looked at this issue even five years ago. But now is the time to leverage those prior investments and get an answer."[17]

Susan G. Komen for the Cure has funded a number of innovative studies, including one conducted by researchers at the Dana-Farber Cancer Institute that could potentially lead to a drug to prevent or treat BRCA-associated breast cancers.[18] Ordinarily, normal cells have a backup repair system for cells with DNA errors. When the BRCA mutation is present, however, the cells can co-opt that system to their advantage, making it possible for cancer to develop. Novel agents called PARP inhibitors, currently being tested in animals, may be able to block the backup DNA repair pathways, causing sufficient harm to cancer cells so that they self-destruct without damaging normal cells.

The Avon Foundation's Breast Cancer Crusade is on the trail of an easy-to-obtain early marker of breast cancer. In recent years, the foundation has invested more than $25 million in primary prevention research, including the search for markers in the blood or saliva or in substances originating directly from the breast, such as nipple discharges or breast milk.[19] "That would be more practical and more promising for detection," says Marc Hurlbert, PhD, the executive director of breast cancer programs of the Avon Foundation for Women and the Avon Breast Cancer Crusade. "When you go to saliva or blood to find a marker for breast cancer, it is more challenging, but we are not giving up."

The Dr. Susan Love Research Foundation, which has the goal of eradicating breast cancer, focuses especially on research on the breast ducts, where cancer begins. Its founder—author of the "bible" in the field, *Dr. Susan Love's Breast Book*—is a leading advocate, clinician, and researcher. With grants totaling more than $900,000 over an 8-year period, the foundation has helped to jump-start innovative research, allowing investigators to leverage additional funds from other sources.

The foundation has also created the Army of Women Program, with funding from the Avon Foundation for Women, to build a base of volunteers willing to participate in breast cancer research. Depending on the study, participants may be asked to complete surveys or provide samples of blood, urine, saliva, breast fluid, or breast tissue in order to help researchers test new markers for the detection, prevention, or treatment of breast cancer.

The Breast Cancer Research Foundation is funding studies of the links among obesity, inflammation of the breast, hormone levels, and cancer. For example, Dr. Clifford Hudis, chief of the Breast Cancer Medicine Service at Memorial Sloan-Kettering Cancer Center, and his colleague Andrew Dannenberg, MD, director of the Weill Cornell Cancer Center, New York, have created an "inflammatory index" to measure lesions found in the breasts of obese women. Their goal is to determine whether obesity-related breast inflammation is a risk factor for breast cancer and how best to modify it.[20]

The Lustgarten Foundation has taken the lead in funding private research to find ways to prevent and treat pancreatic cancer. Six world-renowned institutions are working collaboratively through the foundation's Pancreatic Cancer Research Consortium. In 2008, a team led by Bert Vogelstein, MD, director of the Ludwig Center for Cancer Genetics and Therapeutics at Johns Hopkins School of Medicine and a science advisor at Lustgarten, completed a map of the genetic structure of pancreatic cancer, sequencing 20,000 genes. The team found an average of 63 mutations in each of the 24 discrete types of pancreatic cancers. Dr. Vogelstein says the blueprint could lead to diagnostic tests for very early-stage disease. "We hope that in a number of years, say 10 years, every person over 50 on their routine yearly health exam will be able to get a blood test or an imaging test that will involve the detection of very early cancers when they can still be cured either surgically or perhaps just through fiber optic surgery."[21]

The Lung Cancer Research Foundation (LCRF) looks for advances in basic science that might have implications for patient care. "Over the past decade, there has been an explosion in lung research and our understanding of the disease," says Laurie C. Carson, the foundation's founder and president. "I'd like to see that information translated into clinical treatments."

Several university-based programs funded by Susan G. Komen for the Cure are also conducting promising research. At Duke University, scientists are trying to distinguish lesions (areas of abnormal tissue) contained within the milk ducts that are likely to progress to invasive breast tumors from those that do not pose a threat. If a test can be identified to make that distinction, it is possible that "more than 30,000 women per year may not have to undergo an operation for lesions that have no potential to cause them harm," say the researchers.[22]

Meanwhile, another Komen-funded study at the Mayo Clinic is trying to identify the types and quantities of immune cells in breast tissue with and without cancer.[23] At Fox Chase Cancer Center in Philadelphia, Komen-funded scientists are working to identify the active components of hormones generated during pregnancy that appear to protect breast cells.[24]

The Basser Research Center at the University of Pennsylvania was founded in 2012 specifically to study BRCA mutations. Funded by Jon and Mindy Gray to honor Mindy's sister, Faith Basser, who died of ovarian cancer, the research and treatment center has established primary prevention opportunities as a core part of its mission.[25]

In order to personalize treatment, there is a particular effort to distinguish subtypes of cancer and differences between cancerous and noncancerous cells. For example, LCRF-funded researchers at the University of Medicine and Dentistry of New Jersey are studying the pathway of the COX-2 enzyme, which is associated with inflammation, in both cancer and normal cells. MD Anderson Cancer Center scientists funded by LCRF are scrutinizing a protein found in lung cancer patients who have never smoked to see how it might be implicated in cellular damage.[26]

Genetic studies are being employed to improve the detection of colon cancer at a point when it can still be cured easily with surgery. Johns Hopkins' Dr. Bert Vogelstein has identified 140 mutations associated with colon cancer. With funding from the National Colorectal Cancer Research Alliance, he has built on this knowledge to develop a noninvasive test to detect mutations in stool samples. Other groundbreaking work in the field includes the identification of new biomarkers to detect colon polyps, studies of signaling molecules produced by cancer cells, and the search for patterns of proteins in blood samples, which could lead to easier screening techniques.

In a welcome effort to apply existing knowledge, a team at Harvard Medical School funded by the National Colorectal Cancer Research Alliance is studying the best ways to increase colonoscopies in low-income communities. While perhaps not as intriguing as more technical breakthroughs, bringing proven prevention tools to a broader population is every bit as important. The researchers have established a tumor bank that will collect samples from different ethnic groups to determine whether there are significant biological differences in their colon cancers.[27]

Moving Forward

The cutting-edge work in progress across the country is a reassuring reminder that at least some of our resources are dedicated to prevention, early detection, and immunotherapy. We may never be able to cure patients with advanced cancers, even as we try to maintain their quality of life for as long as possible. Our mission is to prevent the trajectory of disease from ever getting started.

THE FINAL WORD

From Imagination to Transformation

W RITING *A WORLD WITHOUT CANCER* HAS been a personal journey of discovery, inspired by the loss of family and friends and informed by an understanding of the way cancer devastates individuals and diminishes society. My experience has strengthened my conviction that there must be a better way to conquer cancer. It has led me to a place where courage and optimism reside.

By now, the billions of dollars spent and the far-too-many years of limited advances should convince us that we will not tame those renegade cells with the familiar approaches we have been using. The disease will find new ways to overcome our most innovative drugs, even those designed to disarm it at a molecular level. Intricate, wily, and tenacious, cancer will not readily release the grip it has on millions of people around the world.

Still, where there is life, there is hope. I have hope that our nation can blaze a new trail in the quest to defeat cancer. We have an urgent need to focus our tremendous financial and intellectual resources on a coordinated and collaborative prevention strategy.

When President Nixon launched a "great crusade against cancer" in 1971, he said that "a long shadow of fear darkens every corner of the earth." So it is today. We need to rekindle the effort to eradicate cancer that began four decades ago.

That must begin with a shared sense of responsibility for making change. As the President's Cancer Panel has said, "our outrage and sorrow about the suffering and loss caused by cancer seem to be felt individually, but not collectively."

With the creation of the National Cancer Prevention Institute (NCPI) I have proposed, we can launch the studies that will make it possible to change that approach. The NCPI will fund researchers to discover new relationships among genetic, environmental, and lifestyle risk factors and the development of cancer. We will learn more about how to target prevention to our individual biological profiles. We will finally turn our attention to studies that tell us such things as how much exposure to chemical contaminants is truly dangerous and what level of a given nutrient each of us needs to gain prevention benefits. Sooner, rather than later, we will develop better screening tools and more vaccines as well.

Across the country, men and women in laboratories, clinics, cancer centers, and private offices labor, mostly invisibly, to stop cancer's relentless march. Along with our respect and admiration, they should be given an opportunity to see themselves as part of something larger. They should understand that they are contributing to a well-coordinated, collaborative model with cancer prevention at its core, and they should be given the resources and support that allow them to be part of that team.

In the stirring "call to action" that closed one of its reports, the President's Cancer Panel left us with this message:

> It is no longer acceptable to say that because cancer is complex, disparities in care are entrenched, and the tobacco companies are powerful, we cannot solve the problem of cancer in America. We can.

To do so, cancer must become a national priority—one that is guided by strong leadership; fueled by adequate funding and productive collaboration among governments, industry, and institutions; and embraced by individuals who understand and accept their personal role in preventing cancer and in demanding meaningful progress.

Anyone who has been touched by cancer, either as a patient or as an involved family member, friend, or colleague, understands the remarkable strength, bravery, and resolve required to fight the disease. Too many of those precious lives have been lost, and others struggle still to overcome a malignant aggressor, aware that cancer has changed their lives forever.

For the sake of Alba, Angela, Bill, Bridget, Carol, Caroline, Charlie, David, Dolores, Don, Ed, Evan, Florence, Giuseppina, Gregg, Irene, Isabel, James, Jeff, Joie, Lynne, Maria, Michael, Mitchell, Nancy, Neil, Nina, Oksana, Penina, Peter, Regina, Richard, Roger, Rosemary, Sheila, Sherry, Susan, Ted, T.J., Toni K., Toni S., and so many others, we must do better.

America has always met challenges with determination and vigor. We can reach our goal to end cancer by combining our vast resources, awesome talents, and tireless energy.

—

This book begins with the stories of some of the cancer patients I have been privileged to know, and so it will end with the story of someone who has lived through cancer. While Caroline experienced great suffering, she won her personal battle with cancer. With a newfound commitment to enjoy life to the fullest, Caroline has allowed this experience to enhance her life, and the lives of others.

Just 23 years old when she felt a surge of intense pain through her left knee, Caroline embarked on a long and brutal trek through the medical system. It began with a misdiagnosis of torn cartilage, which was treated with arthroscopic surgery. Six months later, she finally learned that she had a soft-tissue sarcoma called malignant fibrous histiocytoma.

Caroline underwent months of toxic chemotherapy to shrink the tumor. Then surgeons amputated her entire lower left leg, which led to massive postoperative bleeding and gangrene.

After 18 months of chemotherapy, accompanied by debilitating nausea and seizures, Caroline declared that she was ending her treatment, which had been scheduled to last a full year longer.

"I took my chances that the cancer had been eradicated. It was a bold decision, but I have never experienced a recurrence," she says.

Thirty-five years later, Caroline believes that cancer has helped her to become a more compassionate person. It also inspired her to reconnect with her Catholic faith and to return to school to pursue a master's degree in social work. She now trains volunteers for a breast cancer hotline and counsels patients in need.

Caroline has shared what she calls life's "final precious moments" with far too many cancer patients, a profound and personal connection that has deepened her own appreciation for what matters most. Whether or not they have cancer, many people, including myself, perceive Caroline as a role model. "The thought that my life is being used as a source of inspiration for others is humbling and gratifying," Caroline acknowledges.

Like all of us, Caroline longs for the day when the wisdom and compassion of role models like her do not come from the experience of being a cancer survivor. Her strongest desire is that, as a society, we truly commit to preventing cancer and working together to reach that goal.

Imagine, for a moment, what a transformative, courageous new approach to cancer could look like.

Imagine gathering together everyone with a stake in cancer research and focusing all of our efforts on solutions designed to achieve the greatest results in the least amount of time. Imagine developing vaccines that send cancer into remission forever. Imagine being able to prevent most cancers and to detect those that do occur before they become a real threat. Imagine a world without cancer.

If we fully dedicate ourselves to the prevention of cancer, this impossible dream will become a reality.

NOTES

Chapter 1: Honoring a Commitment

1 National Cancer Act of 1971, National Cancer Institute, http://dtp.nci.nih.gov/timeline/noflash/milestones/M4_Nixon.htm.

2 John F. Kennedy, Rice University, Houston, Texas, September 12, 1962, www.historyplace.com/speeches/jfk-space.htm.

3 *1972 Fact Book,* National Cancer Institute.

4 Ibid.

5 Vincent T. DeVita Jr. and Edward Chu, "A History of Cancer Chemotherapy," Cancer Research 68, no. 21 (2008): 8643–53.

6 The story of Mary Lasker is drawn from "The Mary Lasker Papers," Profiles in Science, National Library of Medicine, http://profiles.nlm.nih.gov/ps/retrieve/Narrative/TL/p-nid/201.

7 National Cancer Attack Act of 1971, House of Representatives Subcommittee on Public Health and Environment Committee on Interstate and Foreign Commerce, Roswell Park Memorial Institute, Buffalo, New York, October 11, 1971, pp. 739–40.

8 Ibid., 760.

9 Ibid., 756.

10 Katherine Harmon, "Is the 'War on Cancer' Winnable? Forty Years after the Unofficial Declaration, the Disease Is Spreading Throughout the Globe," *Scientific American,* March 24, 2011, http://blogs.scientificamerican.com/observations/2011/03/24/is-the-war-on-cancer-winnable-40-years-after-the-unofficial-declaration-the-disease-is-spreading-throughout-the-globe.

11 Scott D. Ramsey, "How Should We Pay the Piper When He's Calling the Tune? On the Long-Term Affordability of Cancer Care in the United States," *Journal of Clinical Oncology* 25 (2007): 175–79.

12 Surveillance, Epidemiology, and End Results (SEER) Stat Fact Sheets, National Cancer Institute, http://seer.cancer.gov/statfacts/html/all.html.

13 Ibid.

14 "A Midpoint Assessment of the American Cancer Society Challenge Goal to Halve the US Cancer Mortality Rates Between the Years 1990 and 2015," *Cancer* 107, no. 2 (2006): 396–405, http://www.ncbi.nlm.nih.gov/pubmed/16770789.

15 Ibid.

16 A *Cancer Incidence and Survival among Children and Adolescents,* 1975–95, SEER, p. 5, http://seer.cancer.gov/publications/childhood/introduction.pdf.

17 "A Midpoint Assessment of the American Cancer Society Challenge Goal to Halve the US Cancer Mortality Rates Between the Years 1990 and 2015," *Cancer* 107, no. 2 (2006): 396–405, http://www.ncbi.nlm.nih.gov/pubmed/16770789.

18 Rebecca *Siegel*, Deepa Naishadham, and Ahmedin Jemal, "Cancer Statistics, 2012," *CA: A Cancer Journal for Clinicians* 62, no. 1 (2012): 10–29.

19 Francis Collins, "Has the Revolution Arrived?" *Nature* 464 (2010): 674–75, http://www.nature.com/nature/journal/v464/n7289/full/464674a.html.

20 Collins, "Has the Revolution Arrived?"

21 "NCI's Varmus Changes the Metaphor: There Is No War on 'Cancer,'" *Medscape* One-on-One interview with Eli Y. Adashi, December 21, 2011, http://www.medscape.com/viewarticle/755368.

22 Ann M. Bode and Zigang Dong, "Cancer Prevention Research—Then and Now," *Nature Reviews Cancer* 9 (2009): 508–16, http://www.ncbi.nlm.nih.gov/pmc/articles/PMC2838238.

23 *Budget Authority by Activity*, National Cancer Institute, http://obf.cancer.gov/financial/attachments/2012cj.pdf.

24 Lester Breslow and William G. Cumberland, "Progress and Objectives in Cancer Control," *Journal of the American Medical Association* 259, no. 11 (1988): 1690–94, http://jama.ama-assn.org/content/259/11/1690.abstract.

25 Ronald B. Herberman, Homer L. Pearce, Scott Lippman, et al., "Cancer Chemoprevention and Cancer Preventive Vaccines—A Call to Action: Leaders of Diverse Stakeholder Groups Present Strategies for Overcoming Multiple Barriers to Meet an Urgent Need," *Cancer Research* 66 (2006): 11540–49, http://cancerres.aacrjournals.org/content/66/24/11540.full.

26 Angela B. Mariotto, K. Robin Yabroff, Yongwu Shao, et al., "Projections of the Costs of Cancer Care in the United States: 2010–2020," *Journal of the National Cancer Institute* 103, no. 2 (2011), 117–28, http://jnci.oxfordjournals.org/content/103/2/117.

27 Graham A. Colditz, Kathleen Y. Wolin, and Sarah Gehlert, "Applying What We Know to Accelerate Cancer Prevention," *Science Translation Medicine* 4 (2012): 127, http://stm.sciencemag.org/content/4/127/127rv4.full.pdf.

28 Siddhartha Mukherjee, *The Emperor of All Maladies* (New York: HarperCollins, 2010), p. 459.

Chapter 2: Understanding Cancer

1 "Harms of Smoking and Health Benefits of Quitting," National Cancer Institute, http://www.cancer.gov/cancertopics/factsheet/Tobacco/cessation.

2 Donna M. Bozzone, *Causes of Cancer* (New York: Chelsea House, 2007), pp. 86–96.

3 "BRCA1 and BRCA2: Cancer Risk and Genetic Testing," National Cancer Institute, http://www.cancer.gov/cancertopics/factsheet/Risk/BRCA.

4 Gary Stix, "Is Chronic Inflammation the Key to Unlocking the Mysteries of Cancer? *Scientific American*, July 2007, republished November 2008, http://www.scientificamerican.com/article.cfm?id=chronic-inflammation-cancer.

5 Seth Raskoff-Nahoum, "Why Cancer and Inflammation?" *Yale Journal of Biology and Medicine* 79 (2006): 123–30.

6 John B. Liao, "Viruses and Human Cancer," *Yale Journal of Biology and Medicine* 79 (2006): 115–22, http://www.ncbi.nlm.nih.gov/pmc/articles/PMC1994798.

7 "Hepatitis Viruses and Cancer Development," CancerQuest, Emory University, http://www.cancerquest.org/hepatitis-virus-cancer.html.

8   "Number of HPV-Associated Cancer Cases Per Year," Centers for Disease Control and Prevention, http://www.cdc.gov/cancer/hpv/statistics/cases.htm.

9   "HPV-Associated Cancer Statistics," Centers for Disease Control and Prevention, http://www.cdc.gov/cancer/hpv/statistics/index.htm.

Chapter 3: The Promise and Limits of Cancer Screening

1   Kimberly K. Vesco, Evelyn P. Whitlock, Michelle Eder, et al., *Screening for Cervical Cancer: A Systematic Evidence Review for the US Preventive Services Task Force* (Rockville, MD: Agency for Healthcare Research and Quality, 2011), http://preview. ncbi.nlm.nih.gov/bookshelf/booktest/br.fcgi?book=es86.

2   "Colorectal Cancer," CDC Vital Signs, www.cdc.gov/vitalsigns/CancerScreening/index.html.

3   Steven H. Woolf and Russell Harris, "The Harms of Screening: New Attention to an Old Concern," *Journal of the American Medical Association* 307, no. 6 (2012): 565–66.

4   James Rafferty and Maria Chorozoglou, "Possible Net Harms of Breast Cancer Screening," *British Medical Journal* no. 343 (2011): d7627, http://www.bmj.com/content/343/bmj.d7627.

5   Otis Brawley, Tim Byers, Amy Chen, et al., "New American Cancer Society Process for Creating Trustworthy Cancer Screening Guidelines," *Journal of the American Medical Association* 306, no. 22 (2011): 2495–99, http://jama.ama-assn.org/content/306/22/2495.full.pdf+html.

6   "SEER Stat Fact Sheets: Prostate," National Cancer Institute, http://seer.cancer.gov/statfacts/html/prost.html.

7   Richard M. Hoffman, S. Noell Stone, David Espey, and Arnold L. Potosky, "Differences between Men with Screening-Detected versus Clinically Diagnosed Prostate Cancers in the USA," *BMC Cancer* 5, no. 27 (2005), http://www.biomedcentral.com/1471-2407/5/27.

8   Allen S. Brett and Richard J. Ablin, "Prostate Cancer Screening: What the US Preventive Services Task Force Left Out," *New England Journal of Medicine* 365, no. 21 (2011): 1949–51, http://www.nejm.org/doi/full/10.1056/NEJMp1112191.

9   Richard J. Ablin, "The Great Prostate Mistake," *New York Times*, March 10, 2010, http://www.nytimes.com/2010/03/10/opinion/10Ablin.html.

10 "Screening for Prostate Cancer: Draft Recommendation Statement," US Preventive Services Task Force, http://www.uspreventiveservicestaskforce.org/uspstf12/prostate/draftrecprostate.htm.

11 "Screening for Prostate Cancer," US Preventive Services Task Force, August 2008, http://www.uspreventiveservicestaskforce.org/uspstf/uspsprca.htm#update.

12 The American Urological Association's guideline on PSA screening is contained in "Prostate-Specific Antigen Best Practice Statement: 2009 Update," http://www.auanet. org/content/guidelines-and-quality-care/clinical-guidelines/main-reports/psa09.pdf. In an October 7, 2011, press release, the association indicated that it was preparing a new clinical guideline: http://www.auanet.org/content/press/press_releases/article. cfm?articleNo=262.

13 "Screening for Breast Cancer: US Preventive Services Task Force Recommendation Statement," *Annals of Internal Medicine* 15, no. 10 (2009): 716–26, http://www. annals.org/content/151/10/716.full#ref-7.

14 National Breast Cancer Coalition, Web pages on mammography screening: http://www. knowbreastcancer.org/controversies/mammography-screening/.

15 John D. Keen and James E. Keen, "What Is the Point: Will Screening Mammography Save My Life? *BMC Medical Informatics and Decision Making* 9, no. 18 (2009), http://www.biomedcentral.com/1472-6947/9/18.

16 H. Gilbert Welch and Brittney A. Frankel, "Likelihood That a Woman with Screen-Detected Breast Cancer Has Had Her 'Life Saved' by That Screening," *Archives of Internal Medicine* 171, no. 22 (2011), pp. E1–E5.

17 Steven Woloshin and Lisa M. Schwartz, "The Benefits and Harms of Mammography Screening: Understanding the Trade-Offs," *Journal of the American Medical Association* 303, no. 2 (2010): 164–65, http://jama.ama-assn.org/content/303/2/164.full#T1.

18 "Screening for Breast Cancer (2002)," US Preventive Services Task Force Recommendation Statement," http://www.uspreventiveservicestaskforce.org/uspstf/uspsbrca2002.htm.

19 "Screening for Breast Cancer: US Preventive Services Task Force Recommendation Statement," *Annals of Internal Medicine* 15 (2009), no. 10: 716–26, http://www.annals.org/content/151/10/716.full.

20 The National Cancer Institute's mammography recommendations are on its Web site: http://www.cancer.gov/cancertopics/factsheet/detection/mammograms.

21 The American Cancer Society's mammography recommendations are on its Web site: http://www.cancer.org/Cancer/BreastCancer/MoreInformation/BreastCancerEarlyDetection/breast-cancer-early-detection-acs-recs. Susan B. Komen for the Cure's recommendations are on its Web site: http://ww5.komen.org/BreastCancer/GeneralRecommendations.html.

22 B. Cady, M. Webb, et al, "Death from breast cancer occurs predominantly in women not participating in mammographic screening." Presentation at the American Society of Clinical Oncology (ASCO) 2209 Breast Cancer Symposium, San Francisco, California, Abstract 24. http://www.asco.org/ascov2/Meetings/Abstracts?&vmview=abst_detail_view&confID=70&abstractID=40559.

23 Robert A. Smith, Stephen W. Duffy, Laszlo Tabar, "Breast Cancer Screening: The Evolving Evidence," *Oncology,* vol. 26, no. 5 (May 15, 2012): 471–486. http://www.cancernetwork.com/breast-cancer/content/article/10165/2070818?pageNumber=3.

24 Heidi D. Nelson, Bernadette Zakher, Amy Cantor, et al., "Risk Factors for Breast Cancer for Women Aged 40 to 49 Years," *Annals of Internal Medicine* 156, no. 9 (May 1, 2012): 635–49.

25 "Cancer Screening—United States, 2010," *Morbidity and Mortality Weekly Report,* January 27, 2012, Centers for Disease Control and Prevention, http://www.cdc.gov/mmwr/pdf/wk/mm6103.pdf.

26 "Cervical Cancer Statistics," Centers for Disease Control and Prevention, http://www.cdc.gov/cancer/cervical/statistics.

27 *Colorectal Cancer Facts and Figures: 2011–2013,* American Cancer Society, http://www.cancer.org/acs/groups/content/@epidemiologysurveilance/documents/document/acspc-028323.pdf.

28 "Cancer Screening—United States, 2010," *Morbidity and Mortality Weekly Report.*

29 American Cancer Society, Cancer Facts and Figures, www.cancer.org/Research/Cancer FactsFigures/index: 18.

30 "The Facts about Lung Cancer," Lung Cancer Foundation of America, http://www.lcfamerica.org/about_lcfa.html.

31 US Preventive Services Task Force, "Lung Cancer Screening," May 2004, http://www.uspreventiveservicestaskforce.org/uspstf/uspslung.htm.

32 Results from the National Cancer Institute's Prostate, Lung, Colon, and Ovary Screening Trial were published in the National Lung Screening Trial Research Team's

"Reduced Lung-Cancer Mortality with Low-Dose Computed Tomographic Screening," *New England Journal of Medicine* 365 (2011): 395–405, http://www.nejm.org/doi/full/10.1056/NEJMoa1102873. More information about the trial is available on the NCI's Web site: http://www.cancer.gov/newscenter/qa/2002/nlstqaQA.

33 The American Cancer Society's recommendations are on its Web site: http://www.cancer.org/Cancer/LungCancer-Non-SmallCell/DetailedGuide/non-small-cell-lung-cancer-detection.

34 Catherine Winters, "The Big O," *Prevention,* September 2011:96.

35 "SEER Stat Fact Sheets: Ovary," National Cancer Institute, http://seer.cancer.gov/statfacts/html/ovary.html.

36 Barbara A. Goff, Lynn S. Mandel, Charles W. Dresher, et al., "Development of an Ovarian Cancer Index: Possibilities for Earlier Detection," *Cancer* 109, no. 2 (2007): 221–27.

37 Anita W. Lim, David Mesher, Aleksandra Gentry-Maharaj, et al., "Predictive Value of Symptoms for Ovarian Cancer: Comparison of Symptoms Reported by Questionnaire, Interview, and General Practitioner Notes," *Journal of the National Cancer Institute* 104, no. 2 (2012): 1–11, http://jnci.oxfordjournals.org/content/early/2012/01/13/jnci.djr486.full; and Ignace Vergote, "Screening for Ovarian Cancer: Not Quite There Yet," *Lancet* 10, no. 4 (2009): 308–9.

38 Winters, "The Big O."

39 Ibid.

40 Saundra S. Buys, Edward Partridge, Amanda Black, et al., "Effect of Screening on Ovarian Cancer Mortality: The Prostate, Lung, Colorectal and Ovarian (PLCO) Cancer Screening Randomized Controlled Trial," *Journal of the American Medical Association* 305, no. 22 (2011): 2295–303.

41 Recommendations against screening for ovarian cancer are included on the Web sites of the American Cancer Society: http://www.cancer.org/Cancer/news/ovarian-cancer-why-screening-isnt-routine; and the National Cancer Institute: http://www.cancer.gov/cancertopics/pdq/screening/ovarian/HealthProfessional/page1.

Chapter 4: Cut, Poison, and Burn: A Look at Today's Treatment Options

1 "Non-Small Cell Lung Cancer Survival Rates by Stage," American Cancer Society, http://www.cancer.org/Cancer/LungCancer-Non-SmallCell/DetailedGuide/non-small-cell-lung-cancer-survival-rates.

2 Julien Geffrelot, F. Toudic Emily, C. Lévy, et al., "Determination of Clear Margin in Breast-Conserving Surgery: Is 1 mm Needed?" *Journal of Clinical Oncology* 28, no. 15, suppl. 515 (2010): 515, http://meeting.ascopubs.org/cgi/content/abstract/28/15_suppl/515.

3 Laurence E. McCahill, Richard M. Single, Erin J. Bowles, et al., "Variability in Reexcision Following Breast Conservation Surgery," *Journal of the American Medical Association* 307, no. 5 (2012), 467–75, http://jama.ama-assn.org/content/307/5/467.full.pdf+html.

4 Bernard Fisher, Stewart Anderson, John Bryant, et al., "Twenty-Year Follow-Up of a Randomized Trial Comparing Total Mastectomy, Lumpectomy, and Lumpectomy plus Irradiation for the Treatment of Invasive Breast Cancer," *New England Journal of Medicine* 347, no. 16 (2002): 1233–41, http://www.nejm.org/doi/full/10.1056/NEJMoa022152.

5 Monica Morrow, "Rational Local Therapy for Breast Cancer," *New England Journal of Medicine* 347 (2002): 1270–1, http://www.nejm.org/doi/full/10.1056/NEJMe020112.

6 Susan M. Love, *Dr. Susan Love's Breast Book,* 5th ed. (Philadelphia: DeCapo Press, 2010), pp. 326, 337.

7 Morrow, "Rational Local Therapy for Breast Cancer."

8 Katherine Harmon, "The Puzzle of Pancreatic Cancer: How Steve Jobs Did Not Beat the Odds—But Nobel Winner Ralph Steinman Did," *Scientific American,* October 7, 2011, http://www.scientificamerican.com/article.cfm?id=pancreatic-cancer-type-jobs.

9 The story of the development of nitrogen mustard as the first cancer chemotherapy and the establishment of the Cancer Chemotherapy National Service Center are described in Vincent T. DeVita Jr. and Edward Chu, "A History of Cancer Chemotherapy," *Cancer Research* 68 (2008): 8643–53, http://cancerres.aacrjournals.org/content/68/21/8643.full.pdf 1.

10 Vincent Koppelmans, Monique M. B. Breteler, Willem Boogerd, et al., "Neuropsychological Performance in Survivors of Breast Cancer More than 20 Years after Adjuvant Chemotherapy," *Journal of Clinical Oncology* 30, no. 10 (2012), http://hwmaint.jco.ascopubs.org/cgi/reprint/JCO.2011.37.0189v1.

11 Scott E. Klewer, Stanley J. Goldberg, Richard L. Donnerstein, et al., "Dobutamine Stress Echocardiography: A Sensitive Indicator of Diminished Myocardial Function in Asymptomatic Doxorubicin-Treated Long-Term Survivors of Childhood Cancer," *Journal of the American College of Cardiology* 19, no. 2 (1992): 394–401, http://www.ncbi.nlm.nih.gov/pubmed/1732369.

12 Sandra M. Swain, Frederick S. Whaley, and Michael S. Ewer, "Congestive Heart Failure in Patients Treated with Doxorubicin: A Retrospective Analysis of Three Trials," *Cancer* 97, no. 11 (2003): 2869–79, http://www.ncbi.nlm.nih.gov/pubmed/12767102.

13 Carmen Phillips, "Chemotherapy Regimen Extends Survival in Advanced Pancreatic Cancer Patients," *National Cancer Institute Cancer Bulletin* 8, no. 10 (2011), http://www.cancer.gov/ncicancerbulletin/051711/page2.

14 The American Cancer Society briefly describes the second cancers caused by treatment on its Web site: http://www.cancer.org/Cancer/CancerCauses/OtherCarcinogens/MedicalTreatments/SecondCancersCausedbyCancerTreatment/second-cancers-caused-by-cancer-treatment-treatments-linked-to-second-cancers.

15 Dawn L. Hershman, Alfred I. Neugut, Judith S. Jacobson, et al., "Acute Myeloid Leukemia or Myelodysplastic Syndrome Following Use of Granulocyte Colony-Stimulating Factors During Breast Cancer Adjuvant Chemotherapy," *Journal of the National Cancer Institute* 99, no. 3 (2007): 196–205, http://www.ncbi.nlm.nih.gov/pubmed/17284714.

16 The early days of targeted therapy are described in V. T. DeVita and E. Chu, "History of Cancer Chemotherapy," *Cancer Research* 2008; 68: 8643–53.

17 Gunter von Minckwitz, Holger Eidtmann, Mahdi Rezai, et al., "Neoadjuvant Chemotherapy and Bevacizumab for HER2-Negative Breast Cancer, *New England Journal of Medicine* 366, no. 4 (2012): 299–309; Harry D. Bear, Gong Tang, Priya Rastogi, et al., "Bevacizumab Added to Neoadjuvant Chemotherapy for Breast Cancer," *New England Journal of Medicine* 366, no. 4 (2012): 310–20; Vishnal Ranpura, Sanjaykumar Hapani, Shenhong Wu, et al., "Treatment-Related Mortality with Bevacizumab in Cancer Patients: A Meta-Analysis," *Journal of the American Medical Association* 305, no. 5 (2011): 487–94, http://www.ncbi.nlm.nih.gov/pubmed/21285426.

18 The safety information on ipilimumab (Yervoy) is at http://www.yervoy.com/patient.aspx.

19 "Gleevec: Questions and Answers," National Cancer Institute, http://www.cancer.gov/newscenter/qa/2001/gleevecqa. Consumer information about imatinib is available on the National Library of Medicine's Web site: www.ncbi.nlm.nih.gov/pubmedhealth/PMH0000345/?report=p.

20 Findings of a normal life expectancy are reported in "CML Patients Taking Imatinib Have Similar Mortality Rates to People in General Population," *Journal of the National Cancer*

Institute 103, no. 7 (2011), http://jnci.oxfordjournals.org/content/early/2011/03/23/jnci.djr127.full.pdf+html.

21 The STAR trial is well described on the National Cancer Institute's Web site: http://www.cancer.gov/clinicaltrials/noteworthy-trials/star/Page1. Study results were published in Victor G. Vogel, Joseph P. Costantino, Lawrence D. Wickerham, et al., for the National Surgical Adjuvant Breast and Bowel Project, "Effects of Tamoxifen vs. Raloxifene on the Risk of Developing Invasive Breast Cancer and Other Disease Outcomes: The NSABP Study of Tamoxifen and Raloxifene (STAR) P-2 Trial," *Journal of the American Medical Association* 295 (2006): 2727–41, http://www.ncbi.nlm.nih.gov/pubmed/16754727. The US Preventive Services Task Force recommendations, "Chemoprevention of Breast Cancer: Summary of the Evidence," are available online: http://www.uspreventiveservicestaskforce.org/3rduspstf/breastchemo/brstchemosum1.htm.

22 The risks of osteoporosis and heart disease are described in Eitan Amir, Bostjan Seruga, Saroj Niraula, et al., "Toxicity of Adjuvant Endocrine Therapy in Postmenopausal Breast Cancer Patients: A Systematic Review and Meta-Analysis," *Journal of the National Cancer Institute* 103, no. 17 (2011): 1299–1309; and Shannon Puhalia, Rachel C. Jankowitz, and Nancy E. Davidson, "Adjuvant Endocrine Therapy for Breast Cancer: Don't Ditch the Switch!," *Journal of the National Cancer Institute* 103, no. 17 (2011): 1280–82.

23 Androgen deprivation therapy is described on the American Cancer Society's Web pages devoted to prostate cancer treatment: http://www.cancer.org/Cancer/ProstateCancer/DetailedGuide/prostate-cancer-treating-hormone-therapy. The potential growth of neuroendocrine cell tumors is described in a November 17, 2011, Weill Cornell Medical College press release: http://weill.cornell.edu/news/releases/wcmc/wcmc_2011/11_17_11.shtml.

24 Early Breast Cancer Trialists' Collaborative Group, "Effect of Radiotherapy after Breast-Conserving Therapy on 10-Year Recurrence and 15-Year Breast Cancer Death: Meta-Analysis of Individualized Patient Data for 10,801 Women in 17 Randomised Trials," *Lancet* 378 (2011): 1707–16, http://www.ncbi.nlm.nih.gov/pubmed/22019144.

25 Early Breast Cancer Trialists' Collaborative Group, "Comparative Effectiveness of Therapies for Clinically Localized Prostate Cancer," Agency for Healthcare Research and Quality, February 5, 2008, http://effectivehealthcare.ahrq.gov/index.cfm/search-for-guides-reviews-and-reports/?pageaction=displayproduct&productid=79#tableb.

26 Juan P. Wisnivesky, Ethan A. Halm, Marcelo Bonomi, et al., "Postoperative Radiotherapy for Elderly Patients with Stage III Lung Cancer," *Cancer,* published online February 8, 2012, http://onlinelibrary.wiley.com/doi/10.1002/cncr.26585/abstract.

27 Andrew Pollack, "Study Raises Concerns about a Faster Radiation Therapy for Breast Cancer," *New York Times,* December 6, 2011, http://www.nytimes.com/2011/12/07/health/research/study-questions-brachytherapy-a-breast-cancer-radiation-treatment.html.

28 Gregory T. Armstrong, Qi Liu, Yutaka Yasui, et al., "Late Mortality among 5-Year Survivors of Childhood Cancer: A Summary from the Childhood Cancer Survivor Study," *Journal of Clinical Oncology* 27, no. 14 (2009): 2328–38, http://www.ncbi.nlm.nih.gov/pmc/articles/PMC2677921.

29 Information on the study of breast cancer risk in survivors of childhood radiation announced at the ASCO June 2012 Meeting can be found at: Mary Elizabeth Dallas, "After Chest Radiation, Girls at Greater Risk for Early Breast Cancer: Study," MedlinePlus, US National Library of Medicine, National Institutes of Health, June 4, 2012. http://www.nlm.nih.gov/medlineplus/news/fullstory_125872.html and Breast Cancer.org "Radiation Therapy to Chest as Child Increases Breast Cancer Risk in Adulthood," http://www.breastcancer.org/risk/new_research/20120605.jsp.

Chapter 5: What the Market Will Bear

1 Jennifer L. Malin, "Wrestling with the High Price of Cancer Care: Should We Control Costs by Individual's Ability to Pay or Society's Willingness to Pay?" *Journal of Clinical Oncology* 28, no. 20 (2011): 3212–14, http://jco.ascopubs.org/content/28/20/3212.full.pdf.

2 Angela B. Mariotto, K. Robin Yabroff, Yongwu Shao, et al., "Projections of the Cost of Cancer Care in the United States: 2010–20," *Journal of the National Cancer Institute* 103, no. 2 (2011), 117–28, http://jnci.oxfordjournals.org/content/103/2/117.

3 Neal J. Meropol and Kevin A. Schulman, "Cost of Cancer Care: Issues and Implications," *Journal of Clinical Oncology* 25 (2007): 180–86, http://jco.ascopubs.org/content/25/2/180.full.

4 Malin, "Wrestling with the High Price of Cancer Care."

5 Tito Fojo, Anne Noonan, and Christine Grady, "How Much Is Life Worth: The Multibillion Dollar Question in Contemporary Oncology," *American Society of Clinical Oncology*, 2011 educational book: 79–81.

6 Scott D. Ramsey, "How Should We Pay the Piper When He's Calling the Tune? On the Long-Term Affordability of Cancer Care in the United States," *Journal of Clinical Oncology* 25 (2007): 175–79, http://jco.ascopubs.org/content/25/2/175.full.

7 *2011 Report: Medicines in Development for Cancer,* Pharmaceutical Research and Manufacturers of America, http://www.phrma.org.

8 Julie M. Donohue, Marisa Cevasco, and Meredith B. Rosenthal, "A Decade of Direct-to-Consumer Advertising of Prescription Drugs," *New England Journal of Medicine* 357 (2007): 673–81, http://www.nejm.org/doi/full/10.1056/NEJMsa070502.

9 "The Impact of Direct-to-Consumer Advertising," FDA, http://www.fda.gov/Drugs/ResourcesForYou/Consumers/ucm143562.htm.

10 Donohue, Cevasco, and Rosenthal, "A Decade of Direct-to-Consumer Advertising."

11 Troyen A. Brennan, David J. Rothman, Linda Blank, et al., "Health Industry Practices That Create Conflicts of Interest: A Policy Proposal for Academic Medical Centers," *Journal of the American Medical Association* 295, no. 4 (2006): 429–33, http://jama.ama-assn.org/content/295/4/429.

12 "Future Pharma: Five Strategies to Accelerate the Transformation of the Pharmaceutical Industry by 2020," KPMG, 2011, http://www.kpmg.com/CH/en/Library/Articles-Publications/Documents/Sectors/pub-20111103-future-pharma-accessible-en.pdf.

13 Joseph A. DeMasi and Henry G. Grabowski, "Economics of New Oncology Drug Development," *Journal of Clinical Oncology* 25, no. 2 (2007): 209–16, http://jco.ascopubs.org/content/25/2/209.abstract.

14 Celgene, 2010 Annual Report, http://ir.celgene.com/phoenix.zhtml?c=111960&p=irol-reportsAnnual.

15 "UT MD Anderson Creates Institute to Accelerate Cancer Drug Development," University of Texas MD Anderson Cancer Center press release, November 11, 2011, http://www.mdanderson.org/newsroom/news-releases/2011/ut-md-anderson-creates-institute-to-accelerate-cancer-drug-development.html.

16 "Profits and Social Responsibility: Chastened Drug Makers Step Up Efforts to Bring Affordable Medicines to Poor Countries," Knowledge@Wharton, February 10, 2011, http://knowledge.wharton.upenn.edu/article.cfm?articleid=2710.

17 John H. Barton and Ezekiel J. Emanuel, "The Patents-Based Pharmaceutical Development Process: Rationale, Problems and Potential Reforms," *Journal of the American Medical Association* 294, no. 16 (2005): 2075–82, http://jama.jamanetwork.com/article.aspx?articleid=201762; and "General Information Concerning Patents," US Patent and

Trademark Office, http://www.uspto.gov/patents/resources/general_info_concerning_patents.jsp#heading-4.

18 Fortune 500 ranking, CNN Money, http://money.cnn.com/magazines/fortune/fortune500/2010/industries/21/index.html.

19 Alex Berenson, "A Cancer Drug Shows Promise, at a Price That Many Can't Pay," *New York Times,* February 15, 2006, http://www.nytimes.com/2006/02/15/business/15drug.html?pagewanted=all.

20 Joan L. Warren, K. Robin Yabroff, Angela Meekins, et al., "Evaluation of Trends in the Cost of Initial Cancer Treatment," *Journal of the National Cancer Institute* 100, no. 12 (2008): 888–97, http://jnci.oxfordjournals.org/content/100/12/888.

21 "Price Negotiation for the Medicare Drug Program: It Is Time to Lower Costs for Seniors," National Committee to Preserve Social Security and Medicare, http://www.ncpssm.org/pdf/price_negotiation_part_d.pdf.

22 Meropol and Schulman, "Cost of Cancer Care."

23 Warren, Yabroff, Meekins, et al., "Evaluation of Trends in the Costs of Initial Cancer Treatment."

24 Mandy L. Gatesman and Thomas J. Smith, "Perspective: The Shortage of Essential Chemotherapy Drugs in the United States," *New England Journal of Medicine* 365 (2011): 1653–55, http://www.nejm.org/doi/full/10.1056/NEJMp1109772.

25 Steven Reinberg, "Cancer Drug Shortages Are Getting Worse, FDA Says," *US News and World Report,* August 24, 2011.

26 Gatesman and Smith, "Perspective."

27 The description of how Medicare reimbursement for chemotherapy has changed, and its impact on prescribing practices, is discussed in Mireille Jacobson, Craig Earle, Mary Price, et al., "How Medicare's Payment Cuts for Cancer Chemotherapy Drugs Changed Patterns of Treatment," *Health Affairs* 29, no. 7, http://content.healthaffairs.org/content/29/7/1391.abstract.

28 Ibid.

29 Ezekiel Emanuel and Victor R. Fuchs, "The Perfect Storm of Overutilization," *Journal of the American Medical Association* 299, no. 13 (2008): 2789–91, http://jama.ama-assn.org/content/299/23/2789.full.pdf+html.

30 Ramsey, "How Should We Pay the Piper When He's Calling the Tune?"

31 Author interview with Dr. John Marshall; and Bret Stetka and John Marshall, "Fighting a Smarter War Against Cancer," *Medscape,* November 17, 2011, http://www.medscape.com/viewarticle/753600.

32 Richard Sullivan, Jeffrey Peppercorn, Karol Sikor, et al., "Delivering Affordable Cancer Care in High-Income Countries: The *Lancet* Oncology Commission," *Lancet* 12 (September-October 2011): 933–80.

33 Peter Gilmore and Surajut Sen, "Dual-Novel Combinations: A New Approach to Competing in the Oncology Marketplace," Oliver Wyman, http://www.oliverwyman.com/media/Dual-Novel_Combination_Drugs.pdf.

Chapter 6: Paying More, Settling for Less

1 Rebecca Siegel, Deepa Naishadham, and Ahmedin Jemal, "Cancer Statistics, 2012," *CA: A Cancer Journal for Clinicians* 62, no. 1 (2012): 10–29.

2 Neal J. Meropol and Kevin A. Schulman, "Cost of Cancer Care: Issues and Implications," *Journal of Clinical Oncology* 25 (2007): 180–86.

3 Ibid.

4 Nancy Walsh, "New Agents for Metastatic Colorectal Cancer Increase Survival, Cost," http://www.medpagetoday.com/HematologyOncology/ColonCancer/19047.

5 Meropol and Schulman, "Cost of Cancer Care: Issues and Implications."

6 Baohui Zhang, Alexi A. Wright, Haiden A. Huskamp, et al., "Health Care Costs in the Last Week of Life," *Archives of Internal Medicine* 169, no. 5 (2009): 480–88, http://archinte.ama-assn.org/cgi/content/full/169/5/480#REF-IOI80189-3.

7 Haiden A. Huskamp, Nancy L. Keating, Jennifer L. Malin, et al., "Discussions with Physicians about Hospice among Patients with Metastatic Lung Cancer," *Archives of Internal Medicine* 169 (2009): 954–62, http://www.ncbi.nlm.nih.gov/pubmed/19468089?dopt=Abstract.

8 Zhang, Wright, Huskamp, et al., "Health Care Costs in the Last Week of Life."

9 Jennifer S. Temel, Joseph A. Greer, Alona Muzikansky, et al., "Early Palliative Care for Patients with Metastatic Non–Small-Cell Lung Cancer," *New England Journal of Medicine* 363, no. 8 (2010): 733–42, http://www.nejm.org/doi/full/10.1056/NEJMoa1000678.

10 Robert Pirker, Jose R Pereira, Aleksandra Szczesna, et al., "Cetuximab plus Chemotherapy in Patients with Advanced Non-Small-Cell Lung Cancer (FLEX) an Open-Label Randomised Phase III Trial," *Lancet* 373, no. 9674 (2009), http://www.ncbi.nlm.nih.gov/pubmed/19410716.

11 Tito Fojo and Christine Grady, "How Much Is Life Worth: Cetuximab, No–Small Cell Lung Cancer, and the $440 Billion Question," *Journal of the National Cancer Institute* 101, no. 15 (June 29, 2009) http://jnci.oxfordjournals.org/content/101/15/1044.full#T1.

12 Ibid.

13 Caroline Robert, Luc Thomas, Igor Bondarenko, et al., "Ipilimumab plus Dacarbazine for Previously Untreated Metastatic Melanoma," *New England Journal of Medicine* 364, no. 26 (2011): 2517–26, http://www.nejm.org/doi/full/10.1056/NEJMoa1104621.

14 Andrew Pollack, "Approval for a Drug That Treats Melanoma," *New York Times,* March 26, 2011.

15 http://www.yervoy.com/patient.aspx.

16 Malcolm J. Moore, David Goldstein, John Hamm, et al., "Erlotinib plus Gemcitabine Compared with Gemcitabine Alone in Patients with Advanced Pancreatic Cancer: A Phase III Trial of the National Cancer Institute of Canada Clinical Trials Group," *Journal of Clinical Oncology* 25, no 15 (2007): 1960–66, http://gidiv.ucsf.edu/course/things/Moore.pdf.

17 Tito Fojo, Anne Noonan, and Christine Grady, "How Much Is Life Worth: The Multibillion Dollar Question in Contemporary Oncology," 2011, American Society of Clinical Oncology educational book: 79–81.

18 "CML Patients Taking Imatinib Have Similar Mortality Rates to People in General Population," *Journal of the National Cancer Institute* 103, no. 7 (2011), http://jnci.oxfordjournals.org/content/103/7/NP.1.full.

19 http://www.breastcancerdeadline2020.org/2020/about-this-deadline.html.

20 *Clinical Cancer Advances 2011: ASCO's Report on Progress Against Cancer,* American Society of Clinical Oncology.

21 Robert A. Burger, Mark F. Brady, Michael A. Bookman, et al., "Incorporation of Bevacizumab in the Primary Treatment of Ovarian Cancer," *New England Journal of Medicine* 365 (2011): 2473–83, http://www.nejm.org/doi/full/10.1056/NEJMoa1104390.

22 Timothy J. Perren, Ann Marie Swart, Jacobus Pfisterer, et al., "A Phase 3 Trial of Bevacizumab in Ovarian Cancer," *New England Journal of Medicine* 365 (2011): 2484–96, http://www.nejm.org/doi/full/10.1056/NEJMoa1103799.

23 Gina Kolata and Andrew Pollack, "Costly Cancer Drug Offers Hope, but Also a Dilemma," *New York Times,* July 6, 2008.

24 "Commissioner Statement: FDA Commissioner Removes Breast Cancer Indication from Avastin Label," FDA, November 18, 2011, http://www.fda.gov/NewsEvents/Newsroom/PressAnnouncements/ucm279485.htm.

25 Kathy Miller, Molin Wang, Julie Gralow, et al., "Paclitaxel plus Bevacizumab versus Paclitaxel Alone for Metastatic Breast Cancer," *New England Journal of Medicine* 357 (2011): 2666–76, http://www.nejm.org/doi/full/10.1056/NEJMoa072113.

26 Gunter von Minckwitz, Holger Eidtmann, Mahdi Rezai, et al., "Neoadjuvant Chemotherapy and Bevacizumab for HER2-Negative Breast Cancer," *New England Journal of Medicine* 366 (2012): 299–309, http://www.nejm.org/doi/full/10.1056/NEJMoa1111065; and Harry D. Bear, Gong Tang, Priya Rastogi, et al., "Bevacizumab Added to Neoadjuvant Chemotherapy for Breast Cancer," *New England Journal of Medicine* 366, no. 4 (2012): 310–20, http://www.nejm.org/doi/full/10.1056/NEJMoa1111097.

27 Alberto J. Montero and Charles Vogel, "Fighting Fire with Fire: Rekindling the Bevacizumab Debate," *New England Journal of Medicine* 366 (2012): 374–75, http://www.nejm.org/doi/full/10.1056/NEJMe1113368.

28 Cori Vanchiere, "National Cancer Act: A Look Back and Forward," *Journal of the National Cancer Institute* 9, no. 5 (2007): 343.

29 Tito Fojo and Christine Grady, "How Much Is Life Worth: Cetuximab, Non-Small Cell Lung Cancer, and the $440 Billion Question," *Journal of the National Cancer Institute* 101, no. 15 (June 29, 2009).

30 Anne Mason, Michael Drummond, Scott Ramsey, et al, "Comparison of Anticancer Drug Coverage Decisions in the United States and United Kingdom: Does the Evidence Support the Rhetoric?" *Journal of Clinical Oncology,* May 24, 2010. http://jco.ascopubs.org/content/early/2010/05/24/JCO.2009.26.2758.abstract

31 "NICE Unable to Endorse New Treatment for Prostate Cancer," NHS, http://www.nice.org.uk/newsroom/pressreleases/CabazitaxelForProstateCancerFAD.jsp.

32 "Final NICE Guidance Published on Bevacizumab for Treating Metastatic Colorectal Cancer," http://www.nice.org.uk/newsroom/pressreleases/FinalNICEGuidance BevacizumabMetastaticColorectalCancer.jsp.

33 "NICE Consults on a New Treatment for Skin Cancer," http://www.nice.org.uk/newsroom/pressreleases/NICEConsultsOnNewTreatmentForSkinCancer.jsp.

34 Bret Stetka and John Marshall, "Fighting a Smarter War Against Cancer," *Medscape,* November 17, 2011, http://www.medscape.com/viewarticle/753600.

Chapter 7: Cancer's Collateral Damage

1 "National Survey of Households Affected by Cancer," USA Today/Kaiser Family Foundation/Harvard School of Public Health Survey Project, http://www.kff.org/kaiserpolls/upload/7591.pdf.

2 Sonya Blesser Streeter, Lee Schwartzberg, Nadia Husain, et al., "Patient and Plan Characteristics Affecting Abandonment of Oral Oncolytic Prescriptions," *Journal of Oncology Practice* 7, no. 3S (2011): 46s–51s, http://jop.ascopubs.org/content/7/3S/46s.full.pdf+html.

3 Didem S.M. Bernard, Stacy L. Farr, and Zhengyi Fang, "National Estimates of Out-of-Pocket Health Care Expenditure Burdens among Nonelderly Adults with Cancer: 2001–2008," *Journal of Clinical Oncology* 29, no. 20 (July 10, 2011):2821–2826. http://jco.ascopubs.org/content/early/2011/05/31/JCO.2010.33.0522.full.pdf+html.

4 Jennifer Malin, "Wrestling with the High Price of Cancer Care: Should We Control

Costs by Individuals' or Society's Willingness to Pay?" *Journal of Clinical Oncology* 28, no. 20 (2010): 3212–13, http://jco.ascopubs.org/content/28/20/3212.full.

5 "When Battling Cancer, Patients Often Face Hefty Expenses," *Kaiser Health News,* October 11, 2011, http://www.kaiserhealthnews.org/features/insuring-your-health/michelle-andrews-on-cancer-patients-hefty-expenses.aspx; and Scott D. Ramsey, Catherine R. Fedorenko, Kyle S. Snell, et al., "Cancer Diagnosis as a Risk Factor for Personal Bankruptcy," *Journal of Clinical Oncology* 29 (2011): http://www.asco.org/ascov2/Meetings/Abstracts?&vmview=abst_detail_view&confID=102&abstractID=82633.

6 Paula Kim, "Cost of Cancer Care: The Patient Perspective," *Journal of Clinical Oncology* 25, no. 2 (2007): 228–32, http://jco.ascopubs.org/content/25/2/228.abstract.

7 Eric Nadler, Ben Eckert, and Peter J. Neumann, "Do Oncologists Believe New Cancer Drugs Offer Good Value?" *Oncologist* 11, no. 2 (2006): 90–95, http://theoncologist.alphamedpress.org/content/11/2/90.full.pdf+html.

8 Deborah Schrag and Morgan Hanger, "Medical Oncologists' Views on Communicating with Patients about Chemotherapy Costs: A Pilot Survey," *Journal of Clinical Oncology* 25, no. 2 (2007): 230–37, http://jco.ascopubs.org/content/25/2/233.full.pdf.

Chapter 8: Shifting the Research Approach

1 The data on health care spending is from the National Health Expenditure Accounts, available on the Centers for Medicare and Medicaid Services Web site: https://www.cms.gov/Research-Statistics-Data-and-Systems/Statistics-Trends-and-Reports/NationalHealthExpendData/NationalHealthAccountsHistorical.html.

2 Sandeep C. Kulkarni, Alison Levin-Rector, Majid Ezzati, et al., "Falling Behind: Life Expectancy in US Counties from 2000 to 2007 in an International Context," *Population Health Metrics* 9, no. 16 (2011): 1–2, http://www.pophealthmetrics.com/content/pdf/1478-7954-9-16.pdf.

3 *National Cancer Institute Budget Authority by Activity,* National Institutes of Health, http://obf.cancer.gov/financial/attachments/2012cj.pdf.

4 A summary of the President's Cancer Panel's February 1, 2011, meeting is at http://deainfo.nci.nih.gov/advisory/pcp/pcp0211/14feb11stmt.pdf.

5 Sharon Begley, "We Fought Cancer . . . and Cancer Won," *Newsweek,* September 5, 2008.

6 Laura Esserman is interviewed on the Web site of The Breast Cancer Research Foundation. http://www.bcrfcure.org/action_meetres_esserman.html.

7 William S. Dalton, Daniel M. Sullivan, Timothy J. Yeatman, and David A. Fenstermacher, "The 2010 Health Care Reform Act: A Potential Opportunity to Advance Cancer Research by Taking Cancer Personally," *Clinical Cancer Research,* December 15, 2010, vol. 16: 5989.

8 Ashish K. Jha, Catherine M. DesRoches, Eric G. Campbell, et al., "Use of Electronic Health Records in U.S. Hospitals," *New England Journal of Medicine* 360 (2009): 1628–38, http://www.nejm.org/doi/full/10.1056/NEJMsa0900592#t=articleTop.

9 The NCI CaBIG story is drawn from an array of other sources, including John T. Foley, "Report Blasts Problem-Plagued Cancer Research Grid," *Information Week,* http://www.informationweek.com/news/government/enterprise-architecture/229401221; Allison Proffitt, "Future Under Review for caBIG and NCI's Informatics Strategy," *Bio-IT World,* March 20, 2012, http://www.bio-itworld.com/2012/03/20/future-under-review-cabig-nci-informatics-strategy.html; and "NCI Bioinformatics after Kenneth Buetow: Varmus Launches Fundamental Redesign," *Cancer Letter,* January 6, 2012, http://cancerletter.wordpress.com/2012/01/06/1. The NCI describes

the goals of caBIG on its Web site: http://cabig.cancer.gov/about. "CaBIG Overview," National Center for Research Resources, May 2006, http://cabig.nci.nih.gov.

10 "An Assessment of the Impact of the NCI Cancer Biomedical Informatics Grid (caBIG): Report of the Board of Scientific Advisors Ad Hoc Working Group," Ad Hoc Working Group on the NCI CaBIG Program, March 2011, http://arc.georgetown.edu/BSAca BIGAssessment.pdf.

11 Sharyl J. Nass, Harold L. Moses, and John Mendelsohn, eds., *A National Cancer Clinical Trials System for the 21st Century: Reinvigorating the NCI Cooperative Group Program*, Committee on Cancer Clinical Trials and the NCI Cooperative Group Program (Washington, DC: National Academies Press, 2010), http://www.nap.edu/catalog.php?record_id=12879.

12 The IOM and the American Society of Clinical Oncology convened a workshop to discuss ways to achieve the aims underlying the IOM recommendations. The report of the workshop, conducted by the American Society of Clinical Oncology and the Institute of Medicine, is *Implementing a National Cancer Clinical Trials System for the 21st Century* (Washington, DC: National Academies Press, 2011), http://books.nap.edu/openbook.php?record_id=13154&page=1.

13 Carmen J. Allegra, J. Milburn Jessup, Mark R. Somerfield, et al., "American Society of Clinical Oncology Provisional Clinical Opinion: Testing for KRAS Gene Mutations in Patients with Metastatic Colorectal Carcinoma to Predict Response to Anti-Epidermal Growth Factor Receptor Monoclonal Antibody Therapy, *Journal of Clinical Oncology* 27 (2009): 2091–96, http://www.ncbi.nlm.nih.gov/pubmed/19188670.

14 The potential harm to colon cancer patients with the K-ras mutation is described in Tito Fojo and David R. Parkinson, "Biologically Targeted Cancer Therapy and Marginal Benefits: Are We Making Too Much of Too Little or Are We Achieving Too Little by Giving Too Much?" *Clinical Cancer Research* 16 (2010): 5972, http://clincancerres.aacrjournals.org/content/16/24/5972.full.

15 Anil Potti, Holly K. Dressman, Andrea Bild, et al., "Genomic Signatures to Guide the Use of Chemotherapeutics," *Nature Medicine* 12 (2006): 1294–1300, http://www.nature.com/nm/journal/v12/n11/full/nm1491.html.

16 Keith A. Baggerly and Kevin R. Coombes, "Deriving Chemosensitivity from Cell Lines: Forensic Bioinformatics and Reproducible Research in High-Throughput Biology," *Annals of Applied Statistics* 3, no. 4 (2009): 1309–24, http://projecteuclid.org/DPubS?service=UI&version=1.0&verb=Display&handle=euclid.aoas/1267453942.

17 A series of articles on the *Medscape* Web site tracked the Duke genomics scandal, including Zosia Chustecka, "Gene-Guided Chemotherapy Research Questions as 3 NCI Trials Are Halted," July 27, 2010, http://www.medscape.com/viewarticle/725844; Roxanne Nelson, "Four Cancer Genomics Papers Retracted from Top Journals," March 4, 2011, http://www.medscape.com/viewarticle/738412; and Roxanne Nelson, "Dr. Potti and Duke University Sue over Faculty Research," September 13, 2011, http://www.medscape.com/viewarticle/749577. The *Economist* also described the case in detail in "An Array of Errors," September 10, 2011, http://www.economist.com/node/21528593.

18 The journal retractions are described on the Web site Retraction Watch: http://retraction watch.wordpress.com/2012/02/06/anil-potti-and-colleagues-retract-ninth-paper-this-one-in-jco.

19 "Evolution of Translational Omics: Lessons Learned and the Path Forward," Institute of Medicine, March 23, 2012, http://www.iom.edu/Reports/2012/Evolution-of-Translational-Omics/Report-Brief.aspx.

20 Roxanne Nelson, "Dr. Potti and Duke University Sue over Faculty Research," September 13, 2011, http://www.medscape.com/viewarticle/749577.

21 Andrew Pollack, "Head of Sloan-Kettering Sued by University of Pennsylvania," *New York Times,* February 22, 2012, http://www.nytimes.com/2012/02/23/business/dr-craig-b-thompson-head-of-sloan-kettering-is-sued.html.

22 "In Legal Brawl, UPenn, Abramson Institute Say Former Director 'Absconded' with Inventions," *Cancer Letter,* March 9, 2012, http://www.cancerletter.com/articles/20120309_2.

23 "UAH Settles Intellectual Property Litigation," University of Alabama, Huntsville, http://www.uah.edu/legal/pdf_files/UAH%20Settles%20Intellectual%20Property%20Litigation.pdf.

24 Bernard Lo, "Serving Two Masters: Conflicts of Interest in Academic Medicine," *New England Journal of Medicine,* Perspective, 362, no. 8 (2010): 669–71, http://www.nejm.org/doi/pdf/10.1056/NEJMp1000213.

25 Bernard Lo and Marilyn J. Field, eds., *Conflict of Interest in Medical Research, Education and Practice,* Committee on Conflict of Interest in Medical Research, Education and Practice, Institute of Medicine (Washington, DC: National Academies Press, 2009), http://www.nap.edu/openbook.php?record_id=12598&page=1.

Chapter 9: The Promise of Prevention

1 Graham A. Colditz, Kathleen Y. Wolin, and Sarah Gehlert, "Applying What We Know to Accelerate Cancer Prevention," *Science Translational Medicine* 4, no. 127 (2012), http://stm.sciencemag.org/content/4/127/127rv4.abstract.

2 The budgets for the National Center for Advancing Translational Science and the Cures Acceleration Network are included in *Fiscal Year 2013: Budget in Brief,* U.S. Department of Health and Human Services, pp. 36–37, http://www.hhs.gov/budget/budget-brief-fy2013.pdf.

3 Colditz, Wolin, and Gehlert, "Applying What We Know to Acclerate Cancer Prevention."

4 David Hemenway, "Why We Don't Spend Enough on Public Health," *New England Journal of Medicine* 362 (2010): 1657–58, http://www.nejm.org/doi/full/10.1056/NEJMp1001784.

5 The research on cancer disparities comes from the American Cancer Society's Web site, http://www.cancer.org/Cancer/news/Features/cancer-disparities-key-statistics; the New York State Department of Health; and numerous journal articles, including Robert Sullivan, Jeffrey Peppercorn, Karol Sikora, et al., "Delivering Affordable Cancer Care in High-Income Countries," *Lancet Oncology* 12, no. 10 (2011): 933–80; Vanessa de Bosset, Julius Atashili, William Miller, and Michael Pignone, "Health Insurance-Related Disparities in Colorectal Cancer Screening in Virginia," *Cancer Epidemiologic Biomarkers Prevention* 17, no. 4 (2008): 834–37, http://www.ncbi.nlm.nih.gov/pubmed/18398024; Tracy Hampton, "Studies Address Racial and Geographic Disparities in Breast Cancer Treatment," *Journal of the American Medical Association* 300, no. 14 (2008), http://jama.ama-assn.org/content/300/14/1641.full; and Adeyinka O. Laiyemo, Chyke Doubeni, Paul F. Pinsky, et al., "Race and Colorectal Cancer Disparities: Health-Care Utilization vs. Different Cancer Susceptibilities," *Journal of the National Cancer Institute* 102, no. 8 (2010): 538–46.

6 President's Cancer Panel, *America's Demographic and Cultural Transformation: Implications for the Cancer Enterprise,* Annual Report, 2009–10, http://deainfo.nci.nih.gov/advisory/pcp/annualReports/pcp09-10rpt/ExecSum.pdf.

7 Ibid.

8 "Policy Basics: Where Do Our Federal Tax Dollars Go?" Center for Budget and Policy Priorities, April 2, 2012, http://www.cbpp.org/cms/index.cfm?fa=view&id=1258.

9 Information about the National Comprehensive Cancer Network is available on its Web site: http://www.nccn.org/about/default.asp.

10 Peter Cram, A. Mark Fendrick, John Inadomi, et al., "The Impact of a Celebrity Promotional Campaign on the Use of Colon Cancer Screening: The Katie Couric Effect," *Archives of Internal Medicine* 163, no. 13 (2003): 1601–5, http://www.ncbi.nlm.nih.gov/pubmed/12860585.

11 "First-Ever Collaborative Summit on Breast Cancer Research Targets New Partnerships and Collaborative Solutions," PR Newswire, November 13, 2007, http://www.redorbit.com/news/health/1142675/firstever_collaborative_summit_on_breast_cancer_research_targets_new_partnerships.

12 President's Cancer Panel, *Reducing Environmental Cancer Risk: What We Can Do Now*, 2008–2009 Report, released April 2010, http://deainfo.nci.nih.gov/advisory/pcp/annualReports/pcp08-09rpt/PCP_Report_08-09_508.pdf.

Chapter 10: Cancer-Proofing the Environment

1 President's Cancer Panel, *Reducing Environmental Cancer Risk: What We Can Do Now*, 2008–2009 Report, released April 2010, http://deainfo.nci.nih.gov/advisory/pcp/annualReports/pcp08-09rpt/PCP_Report_08-09_508.pdf.

2 "Cancer Facts and Figures 2012," American Cancer Society, http://www.cancer.org/acs/groups/content/@epidemiologysurveilance/documents/document/acspc-031941.pdf; and "Fact Sheet: Childhood Cancers," National Cancer Institute, http://www.cancer.gov/cancertopics/factsheet/Sites-Types/childhood.

3 Commission on Life Sciences, *Pesticides in the Diets of Infants and Children* (Washington, DC: National Academies Press, 1993), http://www.nap.edu/openbook.php?record_id=2126&page=1.

4 "Childhood Leukemia, Brain Cancer on the Rise," WebMD Health News, January 26, 2011, http://www.medicinenet.com/script/main/art.asp?articlekey=125152.

5 Sarah Jenkins, Jun Wang, Isam Eltoum, et al., "Chronic Oral Exposure to Bisphenol A Results in a Nonmonotonic Dose Response in Mammary Carcinogenesis and Metastasis in MMTV-erbB2 Mice," *Environmental Health Perspectives* 119, no. 11 (2011), http://ehp03.niehs.nih.gov/article/info%3Adoi%2F10.1289%2Fehp.1103850.

6 "Bisphenol A: Toxic Plastics Chemical in Canned Food: BPA and Human Diseases on the Rise," Environmental Working Group, http://www.ewg.org/node/20937.

7 "Fact Sheet on Perchloroethylene, also known as Tetrachloroethylene," EPA, February 2012, http://epa.gov/oppt/existingchemicals/pubs/perchloroethylene_fact_sheet.html.

8 Among the studies that have found parabens in breast tumors are Lester Barr, George Metaxas, Christopher Harbach, et al., "Measurement of Paraben Concentrations in Human Breast Tissue at Serial Locations across the Breast from Axilla to Sternum," *Journal of Applied Toxicology* 3 (2012): 219–23; and Philippa Darbre and Philip W. Harvey, "Endocrine Disrupters and Human Health: Could Oestrogenic Chemicals in Body Care Cosmetics Adversely Affect Breast Cancer Incidence in Women?" *Journal of Applied Toxicology* 24, no. 3 (2004): 167–76, http://onlinelibrary.wiley.com/doi/10.1002/jat.1358/abstract.

9 "Parabens," FDA, http://www.fda.gov/cosmetics/productandingredientsafety/selectedcosmeticingredients/ucm128042.htm.

10 "Radiation-Emitting Products," FDA, http://www.fda.gov/Radiation-Emitting Products/RadiationSafety/RadiationDoseReduction/ucm199994.htm; and Rebecca Smith-Bindman, "Is Computed Tomography Safe?," *New England Journal of Medicine* 363 (2010): 1–4, http://www.nejm.org/doi/full/10.1056/NEJMp1002530.

11 Martha S. Linet, Thomas L. Slovis, Donald L. Miller, et al., "Cancer Risks Associated with External Radiation from Diagnostic Imaging Procedures," *CA: A Cancer Journal for Clinicians* 62, no. 2 (2012): 75–100, http://onlinelibrary.wiley.com/doi/10.3322/caac.21132/full.

12 "Radiation-Emitting Products," FDA.

13 Amy Berrington de González, Mahadevappa Mahesh, Kwang-Pyo Kim, et al., "Projected Cancer Risks from Computed Tomographic Scans Performed in the United States in 2007," *Archives of Internal Medicine* 169, no. 22 (2009), http://archinte.ama-assn.org/cgi/content/abstract/169/22/2071.

14 "Breast Cancer and the Environment: A Life Course Approach," Institute of Medicine, December 7, 2011, http://www.iom.edu/Reports/2011/Breast-Cancer-and-the-Environment-A-Life-Course-Approach.aspx.

15 Rebecca Smith-Bindman, Jafi Lipson, Ralph Marcus, et al., "Radiation Dose Associated with Common Computed Tomography Examinations and the Associated Lifetime Attributable Risk of Cancer," *Archives of Internal Medicine* 169, no. 22 (2009): 2078–85, http://archinte.ama-assn.org/cgi/content/abstract/169/22/2078.

16 "White Paper: Initiative to Reduce Unnecessary Radiation Exposure from Medical Imaging," FDA, http://www.fda.gov/Radiation-EmittingProducts/RadiationSafety/RadiationDoseReduction/ucm199994.htm.

17 "Breast Cancer and the Environment," Institute of Medicine.

Chapter 11: Ending the Scourge of Tobacco

1 Graham A. Colditz, Kathleen Y. Wolin, and Sarah Gehlert, "Applying What We Know to Accelerate Cancer Prevention," *Science Translational Medicine* 4, no. 127 (2012), http://stm.sciencemag.org/content/4/127/127rv4.abstract.

2 *Surgeon General's Report: The Health Consequences of Smoking,* Centers for Disease Control and Prevention, 2004, http://www.cdc.gov/tobacco/data_statistics/sgr/2004/complete_report/index.htm.

3 Esther K. Wei, Graham A. Colditz, Edward L. Giovannucci, et al., "Cumulative Risk of Colon Cancer up to Age 70 Years by Risk Factor Status Using Data from the Nurses' Health Study," *American Journal of Epidemiology* 170, no. 7 (2009): 863–872, http://aje.oxfordjournals.org/content/170/7/863.full.

4 Michael Eriksen, Judith Mackay, and Hanna Ross, *The Tobacco Atlas,* 4th ed. (Atlanta: American Cancer Society and World Lung Foundation, 2012), http://www.tobacco atlas.org/industry/influence/text.

5 "Adult Cigarette Smoking in the United States: Current Estimate, 2010," Centers for Disease Control and Prevention, http://www.cdc.gov/tobacco/data_statistics/fact_sheets/adult_data/cig_smoking/index.htm.

6 Lydia Saad, "U.S. Smoking Rate Still Coming Down," Gallup Wellbeing, July 24, 2008, http://www.gallup.com/poll/109048/us-smoking-rate-still-coming-down.aspx.

7 "Smoking and Tobacco Use," Centers for Disease Control and Prevention fact sheets, http://www.cdc.gov/tobacco/data_statistics/fact_sheets/index.htm#core10.

8 "Adult Cigarette Smoking in the United States," Centers for Disease Control and Prevention.

9 David A. Kessler, *Question of Intent: A Great American Battle with a Deadly Industry* (New York: Public Affairs, 2001).

10 Elyse R. Park, Sandra J. Japuntich, Nancy A. Rigotti, et al., "A Snapshot of Smokers after Lung and Colorectal Cancer Diagnosis," *Cancer* (2012), http://onlinelibrary.wiley.com/doi/10.1002/cncr.26545/abstract.

11 "Toll of Tobacco in the United States of America," Campaign for Tobacco-Free Kids, May 9, 2012, www.tobaccofreekids.org/research/factsheets/pdf/0072.pdf.

12 *Surgeon General's Report: The 1964 Report on Smoking and Health,* Profiles in Science, National Library of Medicine.

13 *Surgeon General's Report: The Health Consequences of Involuntary Exposure to Tobacco Smoke*, Office on Smoking and Health (US), Atlanta (GA), Centers for Disease Control and Prevention (US), 1986.

14 "Summary of the Master Settlement Agreement (MSA)," Campaign for Tobacco-Free Kids, http://www.tobaccofreekids.org/research/factsheets/pdf/0057.pdf.

15 "Smoking and Tobacco Use: Fast Facts," Centers for Disease Control and Prevention, http://www.cdc.gov/tobacco/data_statistics/fact_sheets/fast_facts.

16 Ibid.

17 "Tobacco Brands Are Targeting Young Blacks," *Advertisement Journal*, April 23, 2012, http://www.advertisementjournal.com/2012/04/tobacco-brands-are-targeting-young-blacks.

18 Eriksen, Mackay, and Ross, *Tobacco Atlas*, p. 62, http://www.tobaccoatlas.org/industry/influence/text.

19 "US Federal Issues," Campaign for Tobacco-Free Kids, http://www.tobaccofreekids.org/what_we_do/federal_issues.

20 "Raising Cigarette Taxes Reduces Smoking, Especially Among Kids (and the Cigarette Companies Know It)," Campaign for Tobacco-Free Kids, http://www.tobaccofreekids.org/research/factsheets/pdf/0146.pdf?utm_source=factsheets_finder&utm_medium=link &utm_campaign=analytics.

21 "State Cigarette Excise Taxes—United States, 2010–2011," Centers for Disease Control and Prevention, March 30, 2012, http://www.cdc.gov/mmwr/preview/mmwrhtml/mm6112a1.htm?s_cid=%20mm6112a1.htm_w.

22 "CDC Report Finds States Lag in Increasing Cigarette Taxes, Undermining Efforts to Reduce Smoking," Campaign for Tobacco-Free Kids, March 29, 2012, http://www.tobaccofreekids.org/press_releases/post/2012_03_29_cdc.

23 "A Broken Promise to Our Children: The 1998 State Tobacco Settlement 13 Years Later," Robert Wood Johnson Foundation, November 30, 2011, http://www.rwjf.org/files/research/20111140ctfk.pdf.

24 "Smoke-Free Laws Encourage Smokers to Quit and Discourage Youth from Starting," Campaign for Tobacco-Free Kids, https://www.tobaccofreekids.org/research/factsheets/pdf/0198.pdf.

25 "Smoke-Free Laws," Campaign for Tobacco-Free Kids, http://www.tobaccofreekids.org/what_we_do/state_local/smoke_free_laws.

26 Ellen J. Hahn, "Smokefree Legislation: A Review of Health and Economic Outcomes Research," *American Journal of Preventive Medicine* 39, no. 6, suppl. 1, http://www.ncbi.nlm.nih.gov/pubmed/21074680.

27 "Frequently Asked Questions: Final Rule 'Required Warnings for Cigarette Packages and Advertisements,'" US Food and Drug Administration, http://www.fda.gov/Tobacco Products/Labeling/Labeling/CigaretteWarningLabels/ucm259953.htm; and "U.S. Requires Bold New Cigarette Warnings," Campaign for Tobacco-Free Kids, http://www.tobaccofreekids.org/what_we_do/federal_issues/graphic_warning_labels.

Chapter 12: Fighting Cancer with Nutrition and Physical Activity

1 Graham A. Colditz, Kathleen Y. Wolin, and Sarah Gehlert, "Applying What We Know to Accelerate Cancer Prevention," *Science Translational Medicine* 4, no. 127 (2012), http://stm.sciencemag.org/content/4/127/127rv4.full.pdf.

2 Eugenia E. Calle, Carmen Rodriguez, Kimberly Walker-Thurmond, and Michael J. Thun, "Overweight, Obesity and Mortality from Cancer in a Prospectively Studied Cohort of U.S. Adults," *New England Journal of Medicine* 348 (2003): 1625–38, http://www.nejm.org/doi/full/10.1056/NEJMoa021423.

3 "U.S. Obesity Trends," Centers for Disease Control and Prevention, http://www.cdc.gov/obesity/data/trends.html.

4 Sonia S. Maruti, Walter C. Willett, Diane Feskanich, et al., "A Prospective Study of Age-Specific Physical Activity and Premenopausal Breast Cancer," *Journal of the National Cancer Institute* 1000, no. 10 (2008): 728–37, http://jnci.oxfordjournals.org/content/100/10/728.full.pdf+html.

5 I-Min Lee, "Physical Activity and Cancer Prevention: Data from Epidemiologic Studies," *Medicine and Science in Sports and Exercise* 35, no. 11 (2003): 1823–27, http://www.ncbi.nlm.nih.gov/pubmed/14600545.

6 "1988–2008 No Leisure-Time Physical Activity Trend Chart," Centers for Disease Control and Prevention, http://www.cdc.gov/nccdphp/dnpa/physical/stats/leisure_time.htm. The percentage of adults who do not meet the CDC's guidelines for aerobic activity and muscle strengthening is in National Center for Health Statistics, *Health, United States, 2010: With Special Feature on Death and Dying,* Table 70, http://www.cdc.gov/nchs/data/hus/hus10.pdf#070.

7 American Academy of Pediatrics Committee on Environmental Health, "The Built Environment: Designing Communities to Promote Physical Activity in Children," *Pediatrics* 123, no. 6 (2009): 1591–98, http://pediatrics.aappublications.org/content/123/6/1591.full.

8 Amy Winterfeld, Douglas Shinkle, and Larry Morandi, *Promoting Healthy Communities and Reducing Childhood Obesity: Legislative Options,* National Conference of State Legislatures, March 2009, http://www.rwjf.org/files/research/20090330ncsllegislationreport2009.pdf.

9 "Governor Cuomo Launches 'Fresh Connect Farmers' Markets' to Benefit Farmers and Communities Statewide," Governor's Press Office, August 9, 2011, http://www.governor.ny.gov/press/08092011FreshConnect.

10 "Obama Administration Details Healthy Food Financing Initiative," Department of Health and Human Services, press release, February 19, 2010, http://www.hhs.gov/news/press/2010pres/02/20100219a.html.

11 Ron Nixon, "New Rules for School Meals Aim at Reducing Obesity," *New York Times,* January 24, 2012, http://www.nytimes.com/2012/01/26/us/politics/new-school-lunch-rules-aimed-at-reducing-obesity.html.

12 Kelly D. Brownell, Thomas Farley, Walter C. Willett, et al., "The Public Health and Economic Benefits of Taxing Sugar-Sweetened Beverages," *New England Journal of Medicine* 361 (2009): 1599–1605, http://www.nejm.org/doi/full/10.1056/NEJMhpr0905723.

13 "Beverage Companies Market Unhealthy, Sugary Drinks to Children and Teens," Robert Wood Johnson Foundation, http://rwjf.org/childhoodobesity/product.jsp?id=73438.

14 Jonathan Purnell, B.A. Klopfenstein, A.A. Stevens, et al., "Brain Functional Magnetic Resonance Imaging Response to Glucose and Fructose Infusions in Humans," *Diabetes, Obesity and Metabolism* 13, no. 3 (2011): 299–34, http://onlinelibrary.wiley.com/doi/10.1111/j.1463-1326.2010.01340.x/pdf.

15 Miriam E. Bocarsly, Elyse S. Powell, Nicole M. Avena, and Bartley G. Hoebel, "High-Fructose Corn Syrup Causes Characteristics of Obesity in Rats: Increased Body Weight, Body Fat and Triglyceride Levels," *Pharmacology, Biochemistry, and Behavior* 97, no. 1 (2010): 101–6, http://www.ncbi.nlm.nih.gov/pubmed/20219526.

16 Haibo Liu, Danshan Huang, David L. McArthur, et al., "Fructose Induces Transketolase Flux to Promote Pancreatic Cancer Growth, *Cancer Research* 70, no. 15 (2010), http://cancerres.aacrjournals.org/content/70/15/6368.abstract.

17 California Public Interest Group, "Taxpayer Subsidies for Junk Food Wasting Billions,"

September 21, 2011, http://www.calpirg.org/news/cap/taxpayer-subsidies-junk-food-wasting-billions.

18 Jorge Chavarro, Meir Stampfer, Hannia Campos, et al., "A Prospective Study of Blood *Trans* Fatty Acid Levels and Risk of Prostate Cancer," *Proceedings of the American Association of Cancer Research* 47 (2006), http://www.aacrmeetingabstracts.org/cgi/content/abstract/2006/1/943.

19 Véronique Chajès, Anne C.M. Thiébaut, Maxime Rotival, et al., "Association between Serum *Trans*-Monounsaturated Fatty Acids and Breast Cancer Risk in the E3N-EPIC Study," *American Journal of Epidemiology* 167, no. 11 (2008), http://aje.oxfordjournals.org/content/167/11/1312.full.pdf+html.

20 Center for Science in the Public Interest, "Petition for Rulemaking to Revoke the Authority for Industry to Use Partially Hydrogenated Vegetable Oils in Food," May 18, 2004, http://cspinet.org/new/pdf/trans_fat_petition_may_18.pdf.

21 The Center for Science in the Public Interest describes the public health efforts to remove trans fat from the food supply on its Web site: http://www.cspinet.org/transfat.

22 "Policy Statement: Restricting Trans Fatty Acids in the Food Supply," American Public Health Association policy statement, November 6, 2007, http://www.apha.org/advocacy/policy/policysearch/default.htm?id=1366.

23 Hubert W. Vesper, Heather C. Kuiper, Lisa B. Mirel, et al., "Levels of Plasma Trans-Fatty Acids in Non-Hispanic White Adults in the United States in 2000 and 2009," *Journal of the American Medical Association* 307, no. 6 (2012): 562–3.

24 "Non-GMO Shopping Guide," http://www.nongmoshoppingguide.com/about-gmos.html.

25 "Fact Sheet: Genetically Engineered Animals," FDA, http://www.fda.gov/Animal Veterinary/DevelopmentApprovalProcess/GeneticEngineering/GeneticallyEngineered Animals/ucm113597.htm.

26 Reuters, "GMO Salmon: US Consumer Groups Petition FDA for Tougher Probe of Engineered Salmon," Huffington Post, February 7, 2012, http://www.huffingtonpost. com/2012/02/08/gmo-salmon_n_1261536.html.

27 "Genetically Modified Foods," American Academy of Environmental Medicine, http://www.aaemonline.org/gmopost.html.

28 "Eating Cruciferous Vegetables May Improve Breast Cancer Survival," *Science Daily,* April 3, 2012, http://www.sciencedaily.com/releases/2012/04/120403153531.htm.

29 President's Cancer Panel, *Reducing Environmental Cancer Risk: What We Can Do Now, 2008–2009 Annual Report,* http://deainfo.nci.nih.gov/advisory/pcp/annual Reports/pcp08-09rpt/PCP_Report_08-09_508.pdf.

30 International Agency for Cancer Research, World Health Organization, Agents Classified by the IARC Monographs, Volumes 1–105. http://monographs.iarc.fr/ENG/Classification/ClassificationsGroupOrder.pdf.

31 Dagfinn Aune, Doris Chan, Rosa Lau, et al., "Dietary Fibre, Whole Grains, and Risk of Colorectal Cancer: Systematic Review and Dose-Response Meta-Analysis of Prospective Studies," *British Medical Journal* 343 (2011), http://www.bmj.com/content/343/bmj.d6617.

32 Examples of the fiber in foods come from Colorado State University's fact sheet on dietary fiber: http://www.ext.colostate.edu/pubs/foodnut/09333.html.

33 Esteve Fernandez, Liliane Chatenoud, Carlo La Vecchia, et al., "Fish Consumption and Cancer Risk," *American Journal of Clinical Nutrition* 70, no. 1 (1999): 85–90, http://www.ajcn.org/content/70/1/85.full.

34 Harvey J. Murff, Martha J. Shrubsole, Qiuyin Cai, et al., "Dietary Intake of PUFAs and Colorectal Polyp Risk," *American Journal of Clinical Nutrition* 95, no. 3 (2012): 703–12, http://www.ajcn.org/content/95/3/703.full.

35 "Tea and Cancer Prevention: Strengths and Limitations of the Evidence," National Cancer Institute, November 17, 2010, http://www.cancer.gov/cancertopics/factsheet/prevention/tea.

36 Edwina Scott, William P. Steward, Andreas J. Gescher, and Karen Brown, "Resveratrol in Human Cancer Chemoprevention: Choosing the 'Right' Dose," *Molecular Nutrition and Food Research* 56, no. 1 (2011), http://onlinelibrary.wiley.com/doi/10.1002/mnfr.201100400/pdf.

37 R.A. Sharma, A.J. Gescher, and W.P. Steward, "Curcumin: The Story So Far," *European Journal of Cancer* 41, no. 13 (2005): 1955–68, http://www.mendeley.com/research/curcumin-the-story-so-far.

38 "Measuring Biological Response to Curcumin," a clinical trial, is described on the NCI Web site: http://www.cancer.gov/clinicaltrials/featured/trials/ucirvine-uci04-2-02.

39 An Pan, Qui Sun, Adam M. Bernstein, et al., "Red Meat Consumption and Mortality," *Archives of Internal Medicine* 172, no. 7 (2012), http://archinte.ama-assn.org/cgi/content/full/archinternmed.2011.2287.

40 The American Institute for Cancer Research recommendations for cancer prevention are available on its Web site: http://www.aicr.org/reduce-your-cancer-risk/recommendations-for-cancer-prevention/recommendations_05_red_meat.html.

41 Harvard Medical School, "Red Meat and Colon Cancer," March 2008 update, http://www.health.harvard.edu/fhg/updates/Red-meat-and-colon-cancer.shtml.

42 Raphaëlle L. Santarelli, Fabrice Pierre, and Denis E. Corpet, "Processed Meat and Colorectal Cancer: A Review of Epidemiologic and Experimental Evidence," *Nutritional Cancer* 60, no. 2 (2008): 131–44, http://www.ncbi.nlm.nih.gov/pubmed/18444144.

43 Studies of the anticancer agents in food sources are reported on the Web sites of Susan G. Komen for the Cure and the National Colorectal Cancer Research Alliance.

Chapter 13: The Power of Vitamin D

1 Cedric F. Garland, Edward D. Gorham, Sharif B. Mohr, and Frank C. Garland, "Vitamin D for Cancer Prevention: Global Perspective," *Annals of Epidemiology* 19 (2009): 468–83, http://www.cenegenicsfoundation.org/library/library_files/Vitamin_D_for_Cancer_Prevention___Global_Perspective.pdf.

2 Karin B. Michels and Walter C. Willett, "Dietary Factors," in *Principles and Practice of Oncology*, 9th ed., ed. by Vincent T. DeVita Jr., Theodore S. Lawrence, Steven A. Rosenberg, et al. (Philadelphia: Lippincott Williams and Wilkins, 2011).

3 Joan M. Lappe, Dianne Travers-Gustafson, K. Michael Davies, et al., "Vitamin D and Calcium Supplementation Reduces Cancer Risk: Results of a Randomized Trial," *American Journal of Clinical Nutrition* 85 (2007): 1586–91, http://www.ajcn.org/content/85/6/1586.full.pdf+html.

4 The mechanisms by which vitamin D and calcium act against cancer are described in Garland, Gorham, Mohr, and Garland, "Vitamin D for Cancer Prevention: Global Perspective"; and Theresa Shao, Paula Klein, and Michael L. Grossbard, "Vitamin D and Breast Cancer," *Oncologist* 17, no. 1 (2012): 36–45, http://epub.theoncologist.com/i/53740/69.

5 The history of vitamin D as a tool for cancer prevention is described in Sharif B. Mohr, "A Brief History of Vitamin D and Cancer Prevention," *Annals of Epidemiology* 19, no. 2 (2009): 79–83, http://www.sciencedirect.com/science/article/pii/S1047279708003190.

6 Cedric F. Garland, "Do Sunlight and Vitamin D Reduce the Likelihood of Colon Cancer?" *International Journal of Epidemiology* 9, no. 3 (1980): 227–31, http://ije.oxfordjournals.org/content/9/3/227.abstract.

7   Cedric F. Garland, Richard B. Shekelle, Elizabeth Barrett-Connor, et al., "Dietary Vita-
    min D and Calcium and Risk of Colorectal Cancer: A 19-Year Prospective Study in
    Men," *Lancet* 1, no. 8424 (1985): 307–9.

8   Maria V. Grau, John A. Baron, Robert S. Sandler, et al., "Vitamin D, Calcium Supplementation,
    and Colorectal Adenomas: Results of a Randomized Trial," *Journal of the National Cancer
    Institute* 95, no. 23 (2003): 1765–71, http://jnci.oxfordjournals.org/content/95/23/1765.full.

9   Edward D. Gorham, Cedric F. Garland, Frank C. Garland, et al., "Optimal Vitamin D Status
    for Colorectal Cancer Prevention: A Quantitative Meta Analysis," *American Journal of Pre-
    ventive Medicine* 32, no. 3 (2007): 210–16, http://www.ncbi.nlm.nih.gov/pubmed/17296473.

10 Sharif Mohr, Edward Gorham, Alcaraz, et al., "Serum 25-hydroxyvitamin D and
    Breast Cancer in the Military: A Nested Case-Control Study," American Society for
    Nutrition Meetings, April 21 to 25, 2012.

11 Mark J. Bolland, Andrew Grey, Greg D. Gamble, and Ian Reid, "Calcium and Vitamin
    D Supplements and Health Outcomes: A Reanalysis of the Women's Health Initiative
    (WHI) Limited-Access Data Set," *American Journal of Clinical Nutrition* 94, no. 4
    (2011): 1144–49, http://www.ajcn.org/content/94/4/1144.full.pdf+html.

12 Cedric F. Garland, Edward D. Gorham, Sharif B. Mohr, et al., "Vitamin D and Preven-
    tion of Breast Cancer: Pooled Analysis," *Journal of Steroid Biochemistry and Molecu-
    lar Biology* 103, nos. 3–5 (2007): 708–11.

13 Heike Bischoff-Ferrari and Walter Willett, "The Nutrition Source: Comment on the
    IOM Vitamin D and Calcium Recommendations," Harvard School of Public Health,
    http://www.hsph.harvard.edu/nutritionsource/what-should-you-eat/vitamin-d-fracture-
    prevention/index.html#references.

14 B. Dawson-Hughes, A. Mithal, J.-P. Bonjour, et al., "International Osteoporosis Founda-
    tion Position Statement: Vitamin D Recommendations for Older Adults," *Osteoporosis
    International* 21 no. 7 (2010): 1151–54, http://www.ncbi.nlm.nih.gov/pubmed/20422154.

15 "Vitamin D Scientists' Call to Action Statement," GrassrootsHealth, April 2008, http://
    www.grassrootshealth.net/media/download/scientists_letter_072208.pdf; and "Scien-
    tists' Call to D*Action," GrassrootsHealth, http://www.grassrootshealth.net/epidemic.

16 Robert P. Heaney, "Assessing Vitamin D Status," *Current Opinion in Clinical Nutri-
    tion and Metabolic Care* 14, no. 1 (2011), 14: 440–444.

17 VITAL Study (the Vitamin D and Omega-3 Trial), www.vitalstudy.org

Chapter 14: Can Pills Prevent Cancer?

1   Andrew T. Chan, Edward L. Giovannucci, Jeffrey A. Meyerhardt, et al., "Long-Term Use
    of Aspirin and Nonsteroidal Anti-Inflammatory Drugs and Risk of Colorectal Cancer,"
    Journal of the American Medical Association 294, no. 8 (2005), http://jama.ama-assn.
    org/content/294/8/914.full.pdf+html?sid=907bae55-8a1d-44c5-91e9-2b3f96fba683.

2   Peter M. Rothwell, F. Gerald R. Fowkes, Jill F.F. Belch, et al., "Effect of Daily Aspirin
    on Long-Term Risk of Death Due to Cancer: Analysis of Individual Patient Data from
    Randomised Trials," *Lancet* 377, no. 9759 (2011): 31–41, http://www.thelancet.com/
    journals/lancet/article/PIIS0140-6736(10)62110-1/abstract#.

3   Jenny N. Poynter, Stephen B. Gruber, Peter D.R. Higgins, et al., "Statins and the Risk
    of Colorectal Cancer," *New England Journal of Medicine* 352 (2005): 2184–92, http://
    www.nejm.org/doi/full/10.1056/NEJMoa043792.

4   Jaana Kuoppala, Anne Lamminpää, and Eero Pukkala, "Statins and Cancer: A Sys-
    tematic Review and Meta-Analysis," *European Journal of Cancer* 44, no. 15 (2008):
    2122–32, http://www.ejcancer.info/article/S0959-8049%2808%2900498-X/abstract.

5   Crystal Phend, "European Association for the Study of Diabetes: Metformin Still Hot Topic in Cancer Prevention," Medpage, September 27, 2010, http://www.medpage today.com/MeetingCoverage/EASD/22426.

6   Pamela J. Goodwin and Vuk Stambolic, "Metformin, Cancer Risk, and Prognosis," *American Society of Clinical Oncology*, 2011 Educational Book, http://www.asco.org/ ASCOv2/Home/Education%20&%20Training/Educational%20Book/PDF%20Files/ 2011/zds00111000042.PDF.

7   Victor G. Vogel, Joseph P. Costantino, Lawrence Wickerham, et al., "Effects of Tamoxifen vs. Raloxifene on the Risk of Developing Invasive Breast Cancer and Other Disease Outcomes: The NSABP Study of Tamoxifen and Raloxifene (STAR) P-2 Trial," *Journal of the American Medical Association* 295, no. 23 (2006): 2727–41, http://www.ncbi. nlm.nih.gov/pubmed/16754727.

8   The exemestane study, "Exemestane in Preventing Cancer in Postmenopausal Women at Increased Risk of Developing Breast Cancer," is described on the National Cancer Institute clinical trials Web site: http://www.cancer.gov/clinicaltrials/search/view?cdrid =363802&version=healthprofessional.

9   "Exemestane Reduces Breast Cancer Risk in High-Risk Postmenopausal Women," Clinical Trial Results, National Cancer Institute, http://www.cancer.gov/clinicaltrials/ results/summary/2011/exemestane-ASCO0611.

10 Angela M. Cheung, Lianne Tile, Savannah Cardew, et al, "Bone density and structure in healthy postmenopausal women treated with exemestane for the primary prevention of breast cancer: a nested substudy of the MAP.3 randomised controlled trial," *Lancet Oncology* 13, no. 3 (March 2012): 275–84. http://www.thelancet.com/journals/lanonc/ article/PIIS1470-2045(11)70389-8/abstract.

Chapter 15: On the Cutting Edge of Science

1   Shree Bose, "How the Google Science Fair Changed My Life," Huffington Post, March 30, 2012, http://www.huffingtonpost.com/shree-bose/post_2972_b_1388519.html.

2   Carmen Phillips, "FDA Approves First Therapeutic Cancer Vaccine," *NCI Cancer Bulletin* 7, no. 9, May 4, 2010, http://www.cancer.gov/ncicancerbulletin/050410/page2.

3   Marie L. Huber, Laura Haynes, Chris Parker, and Peter Iversen, "Interdisciplinary Critique of Sipuleucel-T as Immunotherapy in Castration-Resistant Prostate Cancer," *Journal of the National Cancer Institute* 104, no. 4 (2012), 273–79, http://jnci.oxford-journals.org/content/early/2012/01/09/jnci.djr514.full.pdf+htm.

4   J. Leonard Lichtenfeld, "Medicare Decides to Pay for Provenge," Dr. Len's Cancer Blog, American Cancer Society, http://www.cancer.org/AboutUs/DrLensBlog/post/ 2011/03/30/Medicare-Decides-To-Pay-For-Provenge-Leaving-The-Battle-Over-Cost-And-Value-To-Be-Fought-Another-Day.aspx.

5   Mahsa Mohebtash, Kwong-Yok Ysang, Ravi A. Madan, et al., "A Pilot Study of MUC-1/ CEA/TRICOM Poxviral-Based Vaccine in Patients with Metastatic Breast and Ovarian Cancer," *Clinical Cancer Research* 17, no. 22 (2011), http://clincancerres.aacrjournals. org/content/early/2011/11/04/1078-0432.CCR-11-0649.short?rss=1.

6   Michael A. Morse, Donna Niedzwiecki, J. Marshall, et al., "Survival Rates among Patients Vaccinated Following Resection of Colorectal Cancer Metastases in a Phase II Randomized Study Compared with Contemporary Controls, *Journal of Clinical Oncology* 29 (2011), http://www.asco.org/ascov2/Meetings/Abstracts?&vmview=abst_detail_ view&confID=102&abstractID=75865.

7   "Novel Brain Tumor Vaccine Acts like Bloodhound to Locate Cancer Cells," Science Daily, January 5, 2012, http://www.sciencedaily.com/releases/2012/01/120105142449.htm.

8   The University of Louisville trial is described on the Lung Cancer Research Foundation Web site: http://www.lungcancerresearchfoundation.org.

9   The University of Pittsburgh Cancer Institute's trial is described on its Web site: http://www.upci.upmc.edu/clinical_research/trialDisplay.cfm?id=4451&type=D.

10 The National Cancer Institute's trials of the *vaccinia* virus to treat liver cancer are described on its Web site: http://www.cancer.gov/clinicaltrials/search/view?cdrid=5828 79&version=HealthProfessional.

11 Information on the University of Minnesota study is available on the Lung Cancer Research Foundation Web site: http://www.lungcancerresearchfoundation.org/research.htm.

12 Details about the National Cancer Institute's Tumor Microenvironment Network are available on its Web site: http://tmen.nci.nih.gov.

13 "The NIH Human Microbiome Project," Genome Research, http://genome.cshlp.org/content/19/12/2317.long

14 Francis S. Collins, *The Language of Life* (New York: HarperCollins, 2010), page 181.

15 The New York University esophageal cancer study is described on the National Institutes of Health Web site: http://projectreporter.nih.gov/project_description.cfm?projectnumber=4UH3CA140233-02.

16 Nancy Zan interview with Jonathan S. Berek, MD, Ovarian Cancer Research Fund, http://www.ocrf.org/index.php?option=com_content&view=article&id=128:an-interview-with-dr-berek-&catid=70:scientific-advisor-blog&Itemid=146.

17 Fran Visco, "Aiming for the Bullseye: A Breast Cancer Vaccine," Huffington Post, March 7, 2012, http://www.huffingtonpost.com/fran-visco/breast-cancer-awareness_b_1327482.html.

18 The Dana-Farber Cancer Institute study is described on the Research Grants (2010 grant) page of the Susan G. Komen for the Cure Web site: http://ww5.komen.org/uploadedFiles/Content/ResearchGrants/GrantPrograms/ResearchGrants/FY10_Research%20Report_Cycle3_7.14.2010.pdf#page=1.

19 The Avon Foundation's research funding is described on its Web site: http://www.avonfoundation.org/breast-cancer-crusade.

20 Clifford Hudis, MD, profile, Breast Cancer Research Foundation, http://bcrfcure.org/action_grantees_hudis.html.

21 "In His Own Words: Dr. Bert Vogelstein Discusses the Pancreatic Cancer Genome Project," Lustgarten Foundation, http://www.lustgarten.org/page.aspx?pid=969.

22 The Duke University research on lesions in the milk ducts is described on the Research Grants (2011 grant) page of the Susan G. Komen for the Cure Web site: http://ww5.komen.org/2011researchgrantspdf/KG110514.pdf.

23 The Mayo Clinic study of immune cells in breast tissue is described on the Research Grants (2011 grant) page of the Susan G. Komen for the Cure Web site: http://ww5.komen.org/2011researchgrantspdf/KG110514.pdf.

24 The studies of hormones generated during pregnancy are described on the Promise Grants page (2010 grant) of the Susan G. Komen for the Cure Foundation Web site: http://ww5.komen.org/uploadedFiles/Content/ResearchGrants/GrantPrograms/ResearchGrants/FY10_Research%20Report_Cycle3_7.14.2010.pdf#page=1.

25 Denise Grady, "Research Center to Focus on Cancer Genes," *New York Times*, May 7, 2012.

26 The lung cancer research activities are described on the Lung Cancer Foundation Web site: http://www.lungcancerresearchfoundation.org/research.htm.

27 The research funded by the National Colorectal Cancer Research Alliance is described on its Web site: http://www.eifoundation.org/programs/eifs-national-colorectal-cancer-research-alliance.

LIST OF EXPERT
INTERVIEWS

THE INDIVIDUALS BELOW INCLUDE EXPERTS IN medicine, research, industry and cancer advocacy who shared their knowledge and insights with me. They have my appreciation for their generous participation.

Carolyn R. Aldigé, president and founder of the Prevent Cancer Foundation

Carole Baggerly, founder and director of GrassrootsHealth and Leader of the D*Action project

Keith A. Baggerly, PhD, professor at the University of Texas MD Anderson Cancer Center's Department of Bioinformatics and Computational Biology

Myra Biblowit, president of The Breast Cancer Research Foundation

Günter Blobel, MD, PhD, John D. Rockefeller Jr. Professor of Cell Biology, investigator at the Howard Hughes Medical Institute, and winner of the 1999 Nobel Prize in Physiology or Medicine

Shree Bose, high school cancer researcher and winner of the 2011 Google Science Fair

Otis Webb Brawley, MD, chief medical officer and executive vice president of the American Cancer Society

Ambassador Nancy G. Brinker, founder and chief executive officer of Susan G. Komen for the Cure

Andrea Califano, PhD, professor of systems biology in the Departments of Biochemistry and Molecular Biophysics and Biomedical Informatics; founding director and chair, Columbia Initiative in Systems Biology; director, Sulzberger Columbia Genome Center, Columbia University Medical Center

Laurie C. Carson, founder and president of the Lung Cancer Research Foundation

Steven K. Clinton, MD, PhD, associate director of the Center for Advanced Functional Foods Research and Entrepreneurship and leader of the Molecular Carcinogenesis and Chemoprevention Program for the Ohio State University Comprehensive Cancer Center

David Cooper, MD, chief executive of Prohealth Care Associates and associate professor at Hofstra Medical School in New York

Andrew Jess Dannenberg, MD, director of Cancer Prevention at New York Presbyterian Hospital-Cornell, director of the Weill Cornell Cancer Center in New York, and the Henry R. Erle, MD-Roberts Family Professor of Medicine

Sarah DeFeo, director of scientific affairs of the Ovarian Cancer Research Fund

Thomas J. Degnan, MD, retired cochief of the Don Monti Division of Hematology/Oncology and retired chairman of the Department of Research of North Shore University Hospital in Manhasset, New York

Eric Ding, PhD, faculty member at Harvard Medical School and Brigham and Women's Hospital, founder and director of the Campaign for Cancer Prevention, and director of Epidemiology for MicroClinics International

James Dougherty, MD, medical and scientific advisor of the Lung Cancer Research Foundation

Carolyn Dresler, MD, MPA, medical director of the Tobacco Prevention and Cessation Program for the Arkansas Department of Health, member of the American Society of Clinical Oncology Prevention Committee, and chair of the Tobacco Control Subcommittee

Ezekiel J. Emanuel, MD, PhD, vice provost for Global Initiatives, chair of the Department of Medical Ethics and Health Policy at the University of Pennsylvania, and Diane v.S. Levy and Robert M. Levy University Professor

Jeff Etchason, MD, senior vice president for Health Systems Research and Innovation at the Lehigh Valley Health Network

Tito Fojo, MD, PhD, program director of medical oncology and head of the Experimental Therapeutics Section at the National Cancer Institute

Cedric Frank Garland, DrPH, FACE, professor of family and preventive medicine (epidemiology), member of the Moores Cancer Center of the University of California San Diego, and cofounder of the D*Action project.

Paul Goldberg, publisher and editor of *The Cancer Letter*

James L. Gulley, MD, PhD, FACP, director of the Clinical Trials Group in the Laboratory of Tumor Immunology and Biology at the National Cancer

Institute and senior staff clinician in the Medical Oncology Branch of the Center for Cancer Research, also at the National Cancer Institute

Robert P. Heaney, MD, John A. Creighton University Professor at Creighton University

Ronald Herberman, MD, chief medical officer of the Intrexon Corporation in Germantown, Maryland, and former director of the University of Pittsburgh Cancer Institute

Clifford Hudis, MD, chief of the Breast Cancer Program at Memorial Sloan-Kettering Cancer Center and incoming president of the American Society of Clinical Oncology for 2013-2014

Marc Hurlbert, PhD, executive director of global breast cancer programs of the Avon Foundation for Women and the Avon Breast Cancer Crusade

James Holland, MD, distinguished professor of neoplastic diseases at Mt. Sinai Hospital in New York

Constantine Kaniklidis, director of medical research of the No Surrender Breast Cancer Foundation (NSBCF)

Kerri Kaplan, executive director of the Lustgarten Foundation

Barnett Kramer, MD, MPH, director of the Division of Prevention at the National Cancer Institute

Scott Lipkin, DPM, chief of the Network Office of Research and Innovation at the Lehigh Valley Health Network

Kathleen Lobb, senior vice-president of communications for the Entertainment Industry Foundation's National Colorectal Cancer Research Alliance

John L. Marshall, MD, professor of medicine, chief of the Division of Hematology/Oncology, and director of Clinical Research at the Lombardi Comprehensive Cancer Center at Georgetown University in Washington, DC

Tony Martell, founder of the T.J. Martell Foundation

Margaret Mastrianni, deputy director and principal liaison for Scientific Advisors and Grants at The Breast Cancer Research Foundation

Jill Fishbane-Mayer, MD, gynecologist in private practice in New York City and assistant attending of Obstetrics, Gynecology, and Reproductive Science at Mount Sinai Hospital

Maria K. Mitchell, PhD, founder and president of AMDeC

Julie Mitnick, MD, radiologist, founder of Murray Hill Radiology, and associate professor of clinical radiology at New York University School of Medicine

Suresh Mohla, PhD, project director of the Tumor Microenvironment Network and chief of the Tumor Biology and Metastasis Branch in the Division of Cancer Biology at the National Cancer Institute

Saresh Nair, MD, senior medical director of Medical Oncology Programs and director of oncology research at the Lehigh Valley Health Network

Larry Norton, MD, deputy physician-in-chief of the Breast Cancer Program at Memorial Sloan–Kettering Cancer Center and chairman of the executive board of scientific advisors at The Breast Cancer Research Foundation

Chandini Portteus, vice president of Research, Evaluation, and Scientific Programs for Susan G. Komen for the Cure

Richard A. Rettig, PhD, former senior social scientist at the RAND Corporation and author of *Cancer Crusade*, the story of the National Cancer Act of 1971

Darrell S. Rigel, MD, founder of Rigel Dermatology, a private practice in New York City, and clinical professor of Dermatology at New York University Medical Center

Caroline Monti Saladino, president of the Don Monti Memorial Research Foundation

Howard Scher, MD, chief of the Genitourinary Oncology Service at the Sidney Kimmel Center for Urologic and Prostate Cancers at Memorial Sloan-Kettering Cancer Center in New York

Nirav R. Shah, MD, MPH, New York State commissioner of health and professor, University at Albany, State University of New York, School of Public Health

Peter Shields, MD, deputy director of the Ohio State University Comprehensive Cancer Center (OSUCCC)

Bruce W. Stillman, PhD, president of Cold Spring Harbor Laboratory

David Sussman, cofounder of the Sussman Family Fund for Breast Cancer Research

Roy Vagelos, MD, retired chairman and CEO of Merck & Co and current chairman of Regeneron Pharmaceuticals and Theravance, two biotechnology companies

Vincent Vinciguerra, MD, chief of the Don Monti Division of Hematology/Oncology, North Shore University Hospital, and professor of medicine of New York University Medical Center

Frances M. Visco, president of the National Breast Cancer Coalition

Nicholas Vogelzang, MD, chair of the American Society of Clinical Oncology Cancer Communications Committee, chair and medical director of the Developmental Therapeutics Committee

Lora Weiselberg, MD, chief of the Breast Cancer Service in the Don Monti Division of Medical Oncology at North Shore University Hospital in Manhasset, New York, and associate professor of medicine at New York University School of Medicine

H. Gilbert Welch, MD, MPH, professor of medicine of the Geisel School of Medicine at Dartmouth, and of Community and Family Medicine at the Dartmouth Institute

Jerome B. Zeldis, MD, PhD, CEO of Celgene Global Health and chief medical officer of Celgene Corporation in Summit, New Jersey

ACKNOWLEDGMENTS

IT IS CLEAR TO ME NOW THAT "IT TAKES A VILLAGE" to write a book about cancer.

The love, patience, and support of my wonderful husband, Howard Maier, and my beautiful daughters, Christina Cuomo Perpignano and Marianna Cuomo Maier, sustained me throughout this journey.

Former secretary of state Madeleine Albright once commented that there is a special place in hell for women who do not help other women. If that is true (and I believe it is!), then Sandra Lee, the Emmy award–winning television host, successful entrepreneur, and generous philanthropist, is assured a place in heaven. My heartfelt gratitude to Sandra for her consistent encouragement, guidance, advocacy, and friendship.

To my brother, Andrew M. Cuomo, thank you for believing in me. Andrew's courageous and visionary leadership as governor of New York State has inspired me.

To my grandparents, Immacolata and Andrea Cuomo, and Mary and Charles Raffa, thank you for showing me how to live a healthful and purposeful life, filled with love.

To my parents, Mario M. Cuomo, "a man for all seasons," and Matilda Raffa Cuomo, thank you for teaching me to serve others and strive for excellence.

My thanks to Maria and Kenneth, Madeline and Brian, Christopher and Cristina, and my wonderful nieces and nephew, Emily, Amanda,

Catherine, Cara, Mariah and Michaela, Samantha, Kristin, Tess, Isabella, Mario, and Carolina for your love and support.

Diane Salvatore, the outstanding editor in chief of *Prevention* magazine, embraced this book from its inception and was committed to its optimal development. Many thanks also to the superb team at Rodale Books, including Stephen Perrine, Trisha Calvo, Nancy Bailey, Maureen Klier, Elissa Altman, Amy DeVito, George Karabotsos, Christopher Rhoads, Danielle Lynn, Aly Mostel, Yelena Nesbit, Brent Gallenberger, Robbie Caploe, Susan Graves, and others for their support, professionalism, and attentiveness. Maria Rodale, the dynamic CEO of Rodale, offered her kind and thoughtful support for this project as did David Zinczenko, EVP, general manager of Rodale's Healthy Living Group. You all have my appreciation and gratitude.

My sincere appreciation for the wisdom, expertise, and advice of Rosalind Lichter, my attorney.

Many thanks for Karyn Feiden's journalistic and editorial skill and her positive attitude.

Thank you to all those friends living with cancer that I've interviewed for the purposes of this book, including Caroline, Joie, Lynne, Sherry, Richard, Susan, and Toni S. Your courage, candor, and generosity are deeply appreciated.

Over the course of several months, I interviewed physicians, researchers, administrators, cancer advocates, and others involved in cancer (see page 272). While each individual is unique, they share common characteristics: their eagerness to share their insights and experiences and their passionate dedication to their missions. While they all have my appreciation, two deserve special mention for their efforts.

Thomas Degnan, MD, my brilliant mentor and loyal friend, has my deepest gratitude for his enthusiastic support of this book. His encyclopedic knowledge, sage advice and good humor are gifts I will treasure forever.

Cedric Garland, DrPH, who has dedicated his life to the study of preventive medicine, generously offered his wisdom and insights, for which I am grateful.

Paul G. Diver has my sincere appreciation for his astute statistical analysis, which enhanced the reporting of data contained in this book. His dedication, patience, and careful attention to detail are extraordinary.

My thanks to Catherine Winters for her editorial expertise and commitment.

The Locust Valley Library has been an invaluable resource to me. The following librarians and staff members have been especially helpful: Leslie Armstrong, Marianne Augustin, Elizabeth Catanzano, Doris DeQuinzio, Camille Farnan, Susan Goldberg, Kathy Jones, Carolyn Oglesby, Sue Ostrowski, Kristine Piana, Marina Ramsay, Kathy Ray, Jennifer Santo, Helga Steele, Trina Stock, Bev Suttie, Michael Vinas, and Deborah Williams. I am truly grateful for their cheerful and efficient assistance.

Debra Rand, MS, AHIP, director for Health Sciences Libraries; Jennifer Boxen, liaison librarian; Nikia Lubin, electronic services coordinator; and June Scarlett, associate dean, all of the Hofstra University North Shore-LIJ School of Medicine, were especially helpful in providing valuable oncology textbooks for my research.

Several individuals at NASA's Office of History are to be thanked for their cooperation and diligence: David Cantor, deputy director; Glenn Bugos, historian; and April Gage, archivist.

Dr. Milton Eisner, of the National Cancer Institute, has my gratitude for his cooperation in providing cancer statistics. Thanks to Lou Gonsalves of the Connecticut Tumor Registry for additional statistical data.

Thanks to two outstanding authors, Rock Brynner (author of *Dark Remedy*) and Richard Rettig (author of *Cancer Crusade*), for sharing their experiences and perspectives. Thanks to Paul Goldberg, editor of *The Cancer Letter,* for his insight and advice.

My gratitude to my book club buddies, Ellen Brous, Jaynne Keyes, Gina Giumarra MacArthur, and Lynne Silver, for their enthusiastic encouragement throughout the creation of this book.

To all those who encouraged me, including Jimmy, James, Kevin and Liz Breslin, Carolyn Smith Bryant, Michael DelGiudice, Jennie and Richard DeScherer, Barbaralee Diamonstein-Spielvogel, Callie Dunn, Ronnie Eldridge, Jon Flaute, Floss and Meyer Frucher, Lynn and Carl Goldstein, Regina Greeven, Kathy and Arthur Hammer, Nancy Hollander, Lorna

Brett Howard, Doug Kelly, Irene and Peter Klein, Angela Giguere Kumble, Gregg Lewis, Margaret Lindner, Joan Maier, Tanya Bastianich Manuali, Richard Marchisotto, Gaetana Marrone-Puglia, Kathy and Joe Mele, Shelby Modell, Caroline Mulcahy, Joseph Murphy, Eve Muscio, Eugene and Liang Nardelli, Carol Opton, Joseph Raffa, Mary Ann Restivo, Louise and Leonard Riggio, Pola and Herman Rosen, Susan Gordon Ryan, Christine Schulze, Aileen Sirey, Richard and Lynda Sirota, Toni and Martin Sosnoff, Kenneth Sunshine, Louis Tallarini, Sherry Thirlby, Patricia Thornton, Mark Vecchio, Vanessa Vecchio, and Joie Wright—your kind words and deeds were more helpful than you may realize.

Special thanks to Arianna Huffington, president and editor in chief of the Huffington Post Media Group and prolific author—a true believer in an integrated approach to good health and in the prevention of diseases. Arianna's enthusiasm for *A World Without Cancer* is appreciated greatly. She has inspired me with her fearless passion for life and joyful energy.

I will always be grateful to the Sisters of Mercy, Sisters of Saint Joseph, and all the other teachers who unselfishly offered me faith and knowledge that have molded and inspired me.

To Mary Ellen Rienzi and Susan Touché—your rigorous artistic and athletic training in dance prepared me to maintain my discipline and focus throughout the course of this demanding project.

And last but certainly not least to Nora Salazar—thank you for your kind and gentle ways, for your encouraging words, and for keeping peace and order in my home during the stormy days and nights.

INDEX